THE PESCATARIAN COOKBOOK FOR BEGINNERS

100 Delicious Simple Seafood Recipes for Healthier Eating Without Skimping on Flavor

50 Air Fryer and 20 Instant Pot recipes included

NATHALIE SEATON

PESCATARIAN COOKBOOK FOR BEGINNERS

© Copyright Nathalie Seaton 2021 - All rights reserved.

The content contained within this book may not be reproduced, duplicated or transmitted without direct written permission from the author or the publisher.

Under no circumstances will any blame or legal responsibility be held against the publisher, or author, for any damages, reparation, or monetary loss due to the information contained within this book. Either directly or indirectly. You are responsible for your own choices, actions, and results.

Legal Notice:

This book is copyright protected. This book is only for personal use. You cannot amend, distribute, sell, use, quote or paraphrase any part, or the content within this book, without the consent of the author or publisher.

Disclaimer Notice:

Please note the information contained within this document is for educational and entertainment purposes only. All effort has been executed to present accurate, up to date, and reliable, complete information. No warranties of any kind are declared or implied. Readers acknowledge that the author is not engaging in the rendering of legal, financial, medical or professional advice. The content within this book has been derived from various sources. Please consult a licensed professional before attempting any techniques outlined in this book.

By reading this document, the reader agrees that under no circumstances is the author responsible for any losses, direct or indirect, which are incurred as a result of the use of the information contained within this document, including, but not limited to, errors, omissions, or inaccuracies.

Table of Contents

- **INTRODUCTION** 8
- **ANCHOVIES** 13
  - #1 Crispy Air-Fried Anchovies (Air Fryer) 13
  - #2 Spanish Style Fried Anchovies (Air Fryer) 15
  - #3 Spaghetti with Capers, Olives, and Anchovies (Pan) 17
- **ATLANTIC CROAKER** 20
  - #4 Korean Spicy Croaker Fish (Air Fryer) 20
  - #5 Marinated Atlantic Croaker (Air Fryer) 22
- **CATFISH** 24
  - #6 Blackened Catfish (Air Fryer) 24
  - #7 Steamed Lemon-Herb Fish (Instant Pot) 26
  - #8 Cajun Fried Fish (Air Fryer) 28
  - #9 Fish Nugget (Air Fryer) 30
- **CRAB** 32
  - #10 Steamed Crab Legs (Instant Pot) 32
  - #11 Crab Bisque (Instant Pot) 34
  - #12 Crab and Corn Chowder (Instant Pot) 36
  - #13 Crab Cakes (Air Fryer) 39
- **FLATFISH** 41
  - #14 Crumbed Fish (Air Fryer) 41
  - #15 Zesty Ranch Fish Fillets (Air Fryer) 43
  - #16 Parmesan Crusted White Fish (Air Fryer) 45
  - #17 Grilled Flatfish with Herb Sauce (Griddle Pan) 47
  - #18 Pan-Fried Sole (Pan) 49
- **HADDOCK** 51
  - #19 Fish and Chips (Air Fryer) 51
  - #20 Haddock in Creamy Tomato Soup (Instant Pot) 53
  - #21 Haddock Pie (Instant Pot) 55
  - #22 Panko Crusted Fried Haddock (Air Fryer) 57
  - #23 Lemon Pepper Haddock (Air Fryer) 59

PESCATARIAN COOKBOOK FOR BEGINNERS

HERRING 61

#24 Oat-Crusted Fried Herring (Air Fryer) 61
#25 Caribbean Fried Smoked Herring (Pan) 63
#26 Fried Herring (Air Fryer) 65
#27 Smoked Salmon and Herring on Toasted Baguette (Oven) 67

LOBSTER 69

#28 Lobster Tails (Instant Pot) 69
#29 Lobster Risotto (Instant Pot) 71
#30 Lobster and Bacon Chowder (Instant Pot) 74
#31 Grilled Lobster with Garlic-Parsley Butter (Griddle Pan) 77

MACKEREL 79

#32 Marinated Mackerel (Griddle Pan) 79
#33 Mackerel Fish Fry (Air Fryer) 81
#34 Fried Crumbed Mackerel (Air Fryer) 83
#35 Fried Mackerel with Ginger Sauce (Pan) 85
#36 Lemon Garlic Mackerel (Griddle Pan) 87
#37 Teriyaki Mackerel (Air Fryer) 89
#38 Honey Soy Mackerel (Air Fryer) 91

MULLET 93

#39 Blackened Mullet (Air Fryer) 93
#40 Mullet with Garlic Oil (Air Fryer) 95
#41 Mullet with Lemon and Caper Sauce (Air Fryer) 97
#42 Mullet with Tomato Sauce (Pan) 99

OYSTERS 101

#43 Oysters with Spicy Butter (Instant Pot) 101
#44 Oyster Stew (Instant Pot) 103
#45 Three-Cheese Baked Oysters (Oven) 105
#46 Air Fried Oysters (Air Fryer) 107
#47 Breaded Oysters (Air Fryer) 109
#48 Almond and Cheese Crusted Oysters (Air Fryer) 111

POLLOCK 113

#49 Coconut Crusted Pollock (Instant Pot) 113
#50 Pollock with Cheesy-Herb Crust (Air Fryer) 116
#51 Crispy Pollock with Tartar Sauce (Air Fryer) 118

#52 Sautéed Pollock with Parmesan Crumbs (Pan) 121
#53 Lemon-Dill Pollock (Air Fryer) 123
#54 Mediterranean Spice Pollock (Air Fryer) 125

SARDINES 127

#55 Lentil and Vegetable Soup with Sardine (Instant Pot) 127
#56 Sweet and Sour Fish (Instant Pot) 129
#57 Mediterranean Sardine Pasta (Pan) 131
#58 Herb-Stuffed Sardines (Air Fryer) 133
#59 Spicy Sardines (Air Fryer) 135
#60 Fried Sardines with Parsley Caper Sauce (Air Fryer) 137

SALMON 139

#61 Salmon Scrambled Eggs (Pan) 139
#62 Teriyaki Salmon (Oven) 141
#63 Fried Salmon with Mustard (Air Fryer) 144
#64 Salmon Cakes (Air Fryer) 146
#65 Honey Glazed Salmon (Air Fryer) 148
#66 Sweet Spicy Salmon (Air Fryer) 150
#67 Balsamic Salmon (Instant Pot) 152
#68 Salmon with Orange Sauce (Instant Pot) 154
#69 Salmon Salad 156
#70 Caramel Salmon (Instant Pot) 157

SCALLOPS 159

#71 Scallops with Lemon-Herb Sauce (Air Fryer) 159
#72 Teriyaki Scallops (Instant Pot) 161
#73 Scallops with Herb Tomato Sauce (Instant Pot) 163

SHRIMP 165

#74 Seafood Gumbo (Instant Pot) 165
#75 Shrimp and Grits (Instant Pot) 168
#76 Shrimp Tacos (Pan) 171
#77 Shrimp Paella (Instant Pot) 173
#78 Shrimp and Broccoli (Instant Pot) 175
#79 Shrimp Fried Rice (Instant Pot) 177
#80 Coconut Shrimp (Air Fryer) 180
#81 Parmesan Shrimp (Air Fryer) 182

PESCATARIAN COOKBOOK FOR BEGINNERS

- #82 Lemon Pepper Shrimp (Air Fryer) 184
- #83 Salt and Pepper Shrimp (Air Fryer) 186

SQUID 188

- #84 Salt and Pepper Squid (Air Fryer) 188
- #85 Squid Stew (Instant Pot) 190
- #86 Squid and Chorizo (Instant Pot) 192

TILAPIA 194

- #87 Fish Sticks (Air Fryer) 194
- #88 Tilapia with Pineapple Salsa (Instant Pot) 196
- #89 Tomato Basil Tilapia (Instant Pot) 198
- #90 Tilapia Fish Curry (Instant Pot) 200
- #91 Lemon Almond Tilapia (Air Fryer) 203

TROUT 205

- #92 Trout with Herb Sauce (Pan) 205
- #93 Mediterranean Flavored Trout (Air Fryer) 207
- #94 Baked Steelhead Trout Fillet (Oven) 209
- #95 Trout with Chimichurri (Air Fryer) 211

TUNA 213

- #96 Tuna Patties (Air Fryer) 213
- #97 Tuna Melt (Air Fryer) 215
- #98 Tuna Casserole (Instant Pot) 217
- #99 Tuna Tacos (Pan) 219
- #100 Tuna Burger (Air Fryer) 221

CONCLUSION 224

NATHALIE SEATON

SPECIAL BONUS!

Want These 2 Bonus books for FREE?

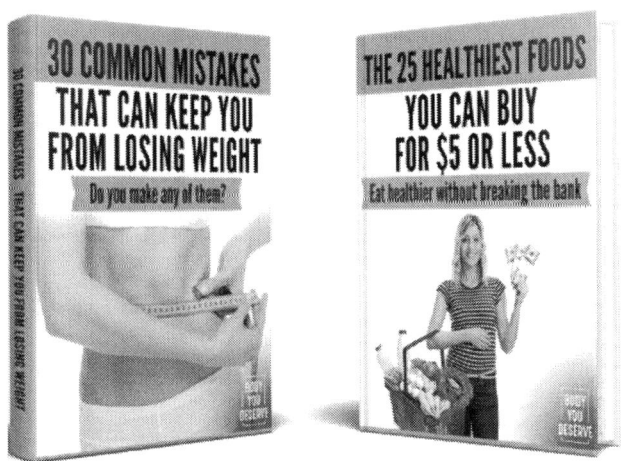

Get **FREE** unlimited access to these and all of our new books by joining our community!

SCAN w/ your camera TO JOIN!

Introduction

A healthy, balanced diet should include at least two portions of fish a week, according to dietitians and nutritionists. Yet, despite advice and recommendations from experts, we often fail to incorporate fish into our diets because it's hard to find simple and delicious fish recipes or the necessary ingredients. I am writing this cookbook to help change that. Adding fish and seafood to your diet will elevate your quality of living with their proven health benefits and nutritional value as well as their rich flavors and recipe variations. Most people live in landlocked areas and haven't had an opportunity to enjoy being near the ocean, much less experiencing the thrill of fishing and handling fresh seafood. I, myself, live in a similar place, but my love for fish and seafood has not been dampened by my environment. You may not have readily available sources of fresh seafood and fish, but you do not need to limit your nutritional choices. Through my experiences, I have learned, and taught others, about resourcing good quality ingredients. More importantly, I have learned to make the most from available ingredients, and I am going to share the results of my hard work through this book.

Are you new to healthy eating and do not know how to do it? Do you want to eat less red meat without compromising on protein? Do you want mouth-watering fish recipes? If your answer is yes, then this ebook is just for you. Whether you enjoy fish or not, the recipes will provide you with the best meaty, umami flavors without being too "fishy." If you do not know how to cook fish, use this book to expand your knowledge in the kitchen and upgrade your palate.

This book has 100 fish and seafood recipes that are easy to make and quick to prepare. Not many people have access to high-grade fish or time to learn and prepare complicated dishes. I have carefully selected and constructed these recipes to use available ingredients and be easily understood, quickly prepared, and, most importantly, delicious to eat.

Seafood and fish have an important role to play in a balanced diet. Sometimes, for healthy eating, people become vegetarian or change their diet, but even those diets are incomplete to an extent. The eating lifestyle often compromises on taste, and dietary supplements are needed to avoid vitamin deficiencies. On the other hand, a pescatarian diet is easier to adopt without compromising flavor or nutrition. According to Merriam-Webster, a pescatarian is "one whose diet includes fish but no other meat." I have no intention to promote pescatarian or any other diet in this book or to limit your food choices. On the contrary, I encourage you to add more variety to your diet by including fish and other seafood meals. Even popular diets, such as the Atkins or the Mediterranean diets promote eating fish two to three times per week.

The benefits of eating fish are endless. It is a source of low-fat, high-quality protein, and it has omega-3 fatty acids. Fish consumption is linked to a decreased risk of heart disease, stroke and death from heart disease. It also develops the fetal vision and nervous system, and it promotes brain health in adults. Fish and seafood are also rich in vitamin D and B2 (riboflavin) and provide minerals, like calcium and phosphorus, among others. The American Heart Association recommends that you should have two meals a week containing fish.

There are many more reasons to eat fish, but some people shy away because they worry about mercury content. Yes, there are some fish high in mercury and should be avoided, such as shark, swordfish, and tilefish. Larger fish usually have more mercury than smaller ones. However, the types of large fish that are high in mercury are not commonly eaten or available. The benefits of having fish in your diet far outweigh any unnecessary concerns about mercury. Fish is even recommended for pregnant women and children for brain development benefits.

Some fish are safer than others to eat. You do not have to worry about that because this recipe book does not include fish with high mercury levels. If you don't know how to make a healthy seafood choice, that's OK. I have organized low-mercury fish into two healthy categories depending on their omega-3 content: "Great Choices" have the most omega-3s, and "Good Choices" have less but are still healthy. The "Great Choices" list includes anchovies, Atlantic mackerel, herring, oysters, Pacific chub mackerel, sardines, shad, trout, and wild or Alaskan salmon (canned or fresh). "Good Choices" include Atlantic croaker, canned light tuna, catfish, crab, flounder and sole (flatfish), haddock, lobster, mullet, pollock, shrimp (wild and most U.S.-farmed), tilapia, scallops, and squid (wild). Continue reading this book to learn more about great and good fish choices how to prepare them efficiently, and how to make great meals with them. After you follow my recipes and instructions, you will have more meal ideas that require very little of your time. This cookbook is also a guide for you to cook terrific dishes like tuna cakes, scrambled eggs with smoked salmon, seared red mullets fillets, marinated mackerel, tacos with shrimp, baked scallops, seafood Thai coconut soup, blackened catfish, and crab boil, to name a few.

Generally, I try my best to avoid all the stress and guesswork for meals after a long day, Like you, I don't want to stand in front of the stove and end up with a bunch of pans and pots. My savior is the Instant Pot, and I love it. You won't believe how easy it is to prepare seafood gumbo or steam crab legs in it. And, the Instant Pot shrimps and grit are out of this world! Nowadays, an air fryer is taking the place of stove-top or oven frying and is trending among health- and fitness-conscious individuals who crave deep-fried foods like onion rings and french fries. This cookbook will give a greaseless option to frying fish and seafood minus the guilt, for example, fish sticks, fish and chips, crumbed fish, breaded sea scallops, and so much more. With this cookbook, there won't be any need to browse the internet aimlessly to find recipes. This recipe book uses the best choices of fish (low mercury and high nutrition) to make uncomplicated, quick-to-make dishes with clear-cut instructions.

With this cookbook, you are ready to start cooking and incorporating fish and seafood into your everyday life. If you do not use the information in this book, then you will miss out on the opportunity to adopt a healthier diet. Once you start preparing these meals, you will save money as well. Homecooked meals are less expensive than the same dish in a restaurant. You will become healthier and happier.

Keep on reading this book to find 100 delicious fish and seafood recipes and unlock many secrets as you go along with your new mindful eating journey.

NATHALIE SEATON

Anchovies

#1 Crispy Air-Fried Anchovies (Air Fryer)

Preparation Time: 10 minutes/Cooking Time: 10 Minutes/Serves: 4 Servings (1/4-pound anchovies per serving)

Nutrition Per Serving: Carbohydrates: 0 grams/Fat: 8 grams/Protein: 28 grams/Fiber: 0 grams/Calories: 189

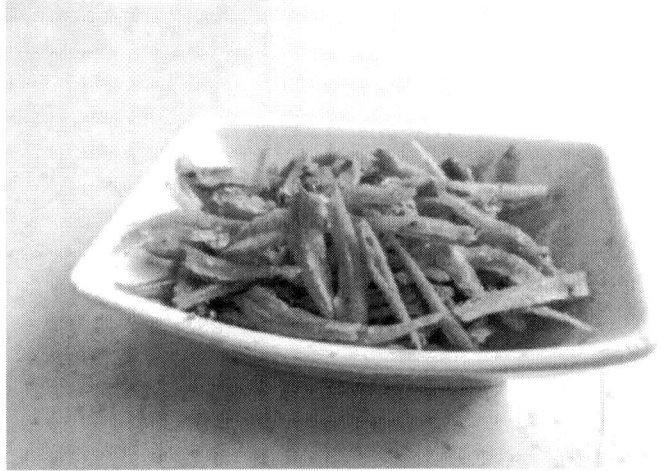

Ingredients

- 1-pound whole anchovies, fresh
- Non-stick cooking oil spray as needed

Directions

1. Prepare the anchovies. Remove its head, tail, and insides, and then place it in a large bowl.
2. Fill the bowl with water. Wash the anchovies around, pour out the dirty water, and then pour in clean water.
3. Spread anchovies on the large plate lined with paper towels, and pat dry with paper towels until completely dry or slightly damp.
4. Switch on the air fryer. Grease its frying basket with oil, insert it into the fryer, close the cover. Select the cooking temperature up to 400 degrees F and preheat.
5. Then spread the anchovies in a single layer in the fryer's basket. Set the frying time to 10 minutes. Let it cook until crisp, stirring anchovies at 7 minutes.
6. Serve immediately or store anchovies in an airtight container for up to 2 months until ready to eat.

#2 Spanish Style Fried Anchovies (Air Fryer)

Preparation Time: 10 minutes/Cooking Time: 30 Minutes/Serves: 4 Servings (1/4-pound anchovies per serving)

Nutrition Per Serving: Carbohydrates: 25.2 grams/Fat: 19.7 grams/Protein: 31.3 grams/Fiber: 1.3 grams/Calories: 405

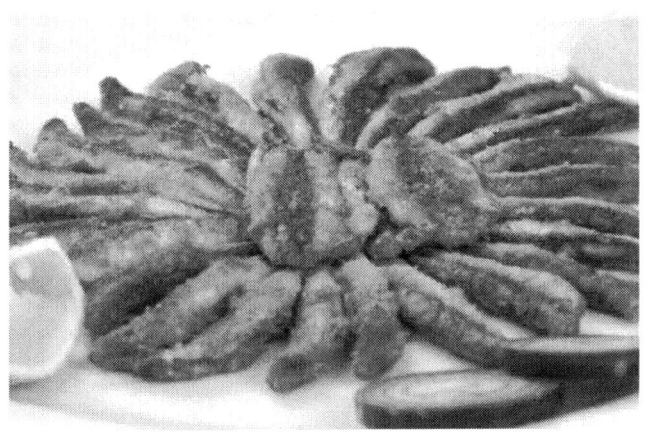

Ingredients

- 1-pound whole anchovies, fresh
- 1 cup all-purpose flour
- 2 teaspoons salt
- non-stick cooking oil spray as needed
- 1 lemon, deseeded, cut into wedges

Directions

1. Prepare the anchovies. Remove its head, tail, and insides and then place in a large bowl.
2. Fill the bowl with water. Wash the anchovies around. Pour out the dirty water, and then pour in clean water.
3. Spread anchovies on the large plate lined with paper towels, and pat dry with paper towels until completely dry or slightly damp.
4. Switch on the air fryer and grease its frying basket with oil. Insert it into the fryer, close the lid, and select the cooking temperature up to 350 degrees F and preheat.
5. Meanwhile, take a shallow dish, place flour in it. Add salt and then stir until mixed.
6. Work on one anchovy at a time, lightly cover it in flour until all sides are coated. Place it on a plate and repeat with the rest.
7. Arrange the prepared anchovies in the fryer's basket, spray it with oil. Set the frying up to 12 minutes, and then let it cook until crisp, turning anchovies at 6 minutes and spraying with oil.
8. Taste the anchovies to adjust salt, and then serve with lemon wedges.

NATHALIE SEATON

#3 Spaghetti with Capers, Olives, and Anchovies (Pan)

Preparation Time: 5 minutes/Cooking Time: 25 Minutes/Serves: 2 Servings (1 pasta bowl per serving)

Nutrition Per Serving: Carbohydrates: 27.9 grams/Fat: 8 grams/Protein: 7.3 grams/Fiber: 3.9 grams/Calories: 203

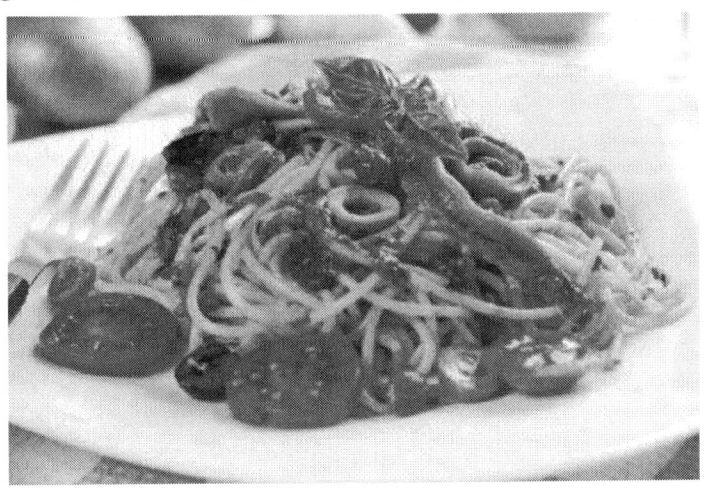

Ingredients

- ½ pound dried spaghetti
- 6 whole anchovy fillets, fresh, cleaned, gutted, meat chopped
- 1 cup whole peeled tomatoes, broken by hands
- ¼ cup chopped pitted black olives
- 1 tablespoon minced garlic

- ¼ cup capers, drained, chopped
- 1 teaspoon salt
- ¼ teaspoon red pepper flakes
- ½ teaspoon ground black pepper
- 6 tablespoons olive oil, divided
- ¼ cup fresh parsley leaves, minced
- 1-ounce grated Parmesan cheese, and more as needed for serving

Directions

1. Take a large skillet pan, fill it half full of water. Stir in a pinch of salt, and then place the pan over high heat.
2. Bring the water to a boil, add spaghetti. Switch heat to a medium-high level. Then cook for 8 to 10 minutes until pasta is firm to the bite (al dente), stirring occasionally. The pasta will be cooked entirely in the sauce. It is best to cook the pasta a minute less than what is indicated on the package.
3. While pasta is cooking, take a medium skillet pan. Place it over medium heat. Then add 4 tablespoons of oil, heat.
4. Add garlic and anchovies into the pan. Stir in red pepper flakes and then cook for 5 minutes until garlic turns golden brown.
5. Add olives and capers. Stir until well blended. Cook for one minute, then stir in tomatoes. Bring the mixture to a boil and continue simmering until the pasta has cooked.

6. When pasta has cooked, remove the pot from heat, reserve a cup of the pasta water, and then drain the pasta through a colander.
7. Add pasta into the tomato sauce, stir in some of the reserved pasta water until the sauce reaches the desired thickness. Cook for one to two minutes until pasta is perfectly softened.
8. Add the remaining oil, minced parsley and cheese. Season with black pepper and a little salt, and then toss until well combined.
9. Divide pasta evenly between bowls and then serve.

PESCATARIAN COOKBOOK FOR BEGINNERS

Atlantic Croaker

#4 Korean Spicy Croaker Fish (Air Fryer)

Preparation Time: 10 minutes/Cooking Time: 10 Minutes/Serves: 3 Servings (2 fish per serving)

Nutrition Per Serving: Carbohydrates: 12 grams/Fat: 1 grams/Protein: 10 grams/Fiber: 1 grams/Calories: 91

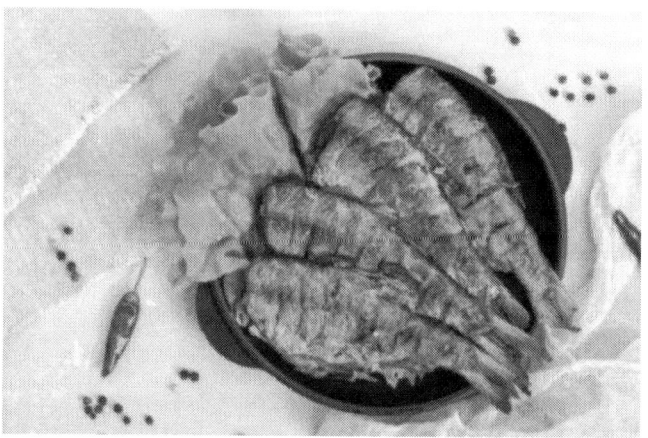

Ingredients

- 6 Atlantic croaker fish, medium-sized, scaled, cleaned
- 1 ½ teaspoon Korean hot pepper paste or any hot pepper paste
- ½ teaspoon soy sauce
- 2 tablespoon honey
- 1 tablespoon rice wine
- Non-stick cooking oil spray as needed

Directions

1. Prepare the fish. Clean and rinse it well, then pat dry with paper towels. Rub the fish with wine and set aside for 5 minutes.
2. In a small bowl, add soy sauce, honey, and hot pepper sauce. Stir until well blended and set aside.
3. Switch on the air fryer. Line the fryer's basket with a foil, and then grease with oil.
4. Insert the fryer's basket into the air fryer and close the cover. Select the cooking temperature up to 400 degrees F and preheat.
5. Make a few cuts on each side of the fish and arrange it in a single layer in the fryer's basket. Brush the top of the fish with honey sauce and then fry for 5 minutes.
6. Flip the fish, brush with the remaining honey sauce and then continue frying for another 5 minutes until done.
7. Serve right away.

#5 Marinated Atlantic Croaker (Air Fryer)

Preparation Time: 20 minutes/Cooking Time: 10 Minutes/Serves: 2 Servings (1 fish per serving)

Nutrition Per Serving: Carbohydrates: 23.8 grams/Fat: 18.9 grams/Protein: 33.7 grams/Fiber: 0.5 grams/Calories: 397

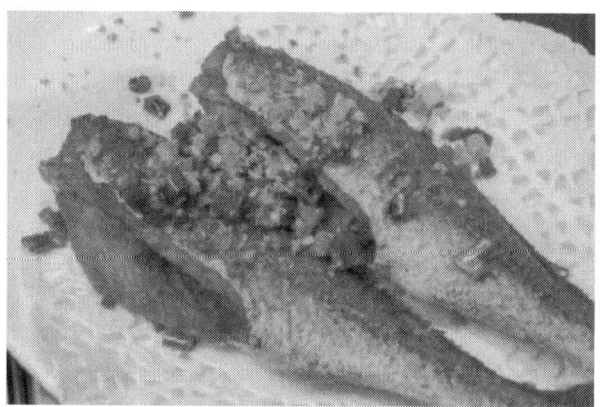

Ingredients

- 2 Atlantic croakers, medium-sized, scaled, cleaned
- 4 tablespoons all-purpose flour
- ½ teaspoon salt
- ¼ teaspoon ground black pepper
- 2 tablespoons minced garlic
- 1 tablespoon corn starch
- 3 tablespoons of rice wine
- Non-stick cooking oil spray as needed

Directions

1. Prepare the fish. Clean and rinse it well. Then dry with paper towels.
2. Take a large bowl, pour in rice wine, add salt, black pepper, and garlic. Stir until mixed.
3. Add fish, toss until coated. Marinate at room temperature for 15 minutes.
4. Meanwhile, take a shallow dish, and place flour in it Add cornstarch and then stir until mixed.
5. Switch on the air fryer and grease the fryer's basket with oil. Close the cover, and then select the cooking temperature up to 400 degrees F and preheat.
6. Arrange a single layer of the marinated fish in the fryer's basket. Spray it with oil. Fry for 10 minutes until done. Flip the other side, spray with oil and fry until thoroughly done.
7. Serve right away.

Catfish

#6 Blackened Catfish (Air Fryer)

Preparation Time: 20 minutes/Cooking Time: 10 Minutes/Serves: 4 Servings (1 fillet per serving)

Nutrition Per Serving: Carbohydrates: 0 grams/Fat: 18 grams/Protein: 22 grams/Fiber: 0 grams/Calories: 251

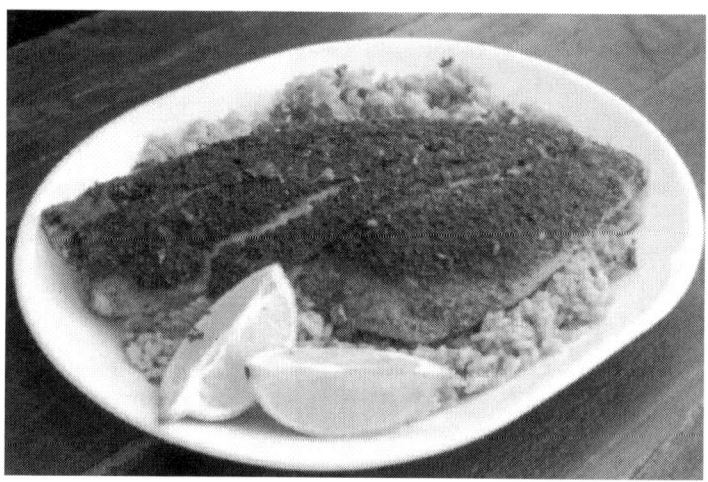

Ingredients

- 4 catfish fillets, skinless, each about 5 ounces
- ¾ teaspoon salt
- ¼ cup fresh parsley
- 1 lemon, cut into wedges
- Non-stick cooking oil spray as needed
  for the Spice Mix:
- ½ cup Cajun seasoning

- 1 tablespoon sweet or smoked sweet paprika
- 1 tablespoon ground black pepper
- 1 teaspoon onion powder
- 1 teaspoon garlic powder
- 1 teaspoon dried oregano
- 1 teaspoon dried thyme or rosemary
- 1/8 teaspoon cayenne pepper

Directions

1. Place all the ingredients for the spice mix in a small bowl. Stir until well mixed.
2. Rinse the fish fillets, and pat dry with paper towels. Sprinkle with salt, let it stand at room temperature for 15 minutes and then drizzle oil over the fillets.
3. Switch on the air fryer, and line the fryer's basket with foil. Grease it with oil.
4. Close the air fryer's cover. Select the cooking temperature up to 400 degrees F and preheat.
5. Meanwhile, sprinkle each of the salted fillets with ¼ cup of the spice mix. Press the spice mix to stick to the fillets. Arrange the fillets in a single layer and place in the fryer's basket.
6. Spray oil over the prepared fillets and close the cover. Fry for 10 minutes until done. Flip the other side, spray with oil and fry until thoroughly cooked.
7. Transfer fried fillets to a plate, sprinkle with parsley, and serve with lemon wedges.

#7 Steamed Lemon-Herb Fish (Instant Pot)

Preparation Time: 10 minutes/Cooking Time: 8 Minutes/Serves: 4 Servings (1 fillet per serving)

Nutrition Per Serving: Carbohydrates: 32 grams/Fat: 4 grams/Protein: 25 grams/Fiber: 4 grams/Calories: 258

Ingredients

- 4 catfish fillets, skinless, each about 5 ounces
- 3 medium potatoes, peeled, thinly sliced
- 1 medium white onion, peeled, sliced into thin rings
- ¼ teaspoon salt
- 1/8 teaspoon ground black pepper
- 4 sprigs of thyme, fresh
- 1 lemon, sliced
- 2 teaspoons olive oil
- 1 ½ cups water

Directions

1. Switch on the 4-quarts instant pot, pour water into the inner pot. Then insert a trivet stand.
2. Place a steamer basket that fits into the inner pot. Line it with a parchment sheet, cover with lemon slices and then layer with fish fillets.
3. Top the fish with onion slices and thyme sprigs. Layer with potato slices. Season with salt and

black pepper. Then drizzle with oil until fully coated.
4. Lower the prepared steamer basket into the trivet stand and close the cover securely.
5. Press the manual button and select the low-pressure setting. The cooking time should be 8 minutes. The instant pot will take 5 to 10 minutes to build pressure, then the cooking timer will start.
6. When the instant pot beeps, quickly release the pressure, and open the instant pot carefully.
7. Serve the fillet right away, or serve it with onion, potato, and lemon slices.

PESCATARIAN COOKBOOK FOR BEGINNERS

#8 Cajun Fried Fish (Air Fryer)

Preparation Time: 5 minutes/Cooking Time: 26 Minutes/Serves: 4 Servings (per serving)

Nutrition Per Serving: Carbohydrates: 0.5 grams/Fat: 15 grams/Protein: 21.1 grams/Fiber: 0.02 grams/Calories: 222.5

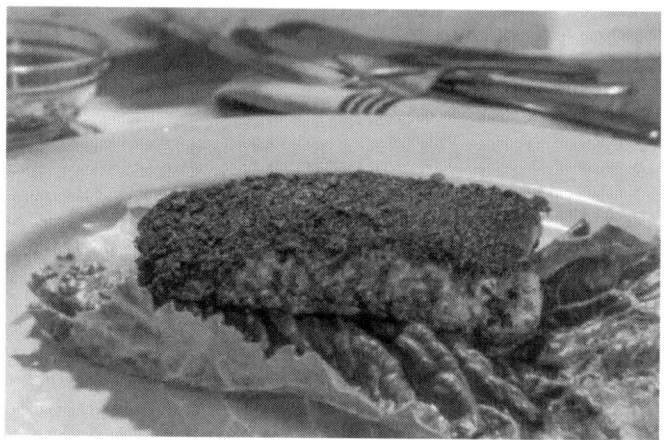

Ingredients

- 4 catfish fillets, skinless, each about 5 ounces
- ¼ cup Cajun seasoning
- 1 tablespoon olive oil
- 1 tablespoon chopped parsley
- Non-stick cooking oil spray

Directions

1. Rinse the fish fillets, and pat dry with paper towels. Sprinkle with Cajun seasoning until fully coated, then drizzle with oil.
2. Switch on the air fryer and grease the fryer's basket with oil. Place it into the fryer and close the cover. Set the cooking temperature up to 400 degrees F and preheat.
3. Arrange the prepared fish fillets in a single layer. Place the fillets in the fryer's basket, spray with oil, and then fry for 10 minutes.
4. Flip each fillet and close the air fryer. Continue frying for 3 minutes until crisp.
5. When done, transfer the fillets to a plate, sprinkle with parsley, and then serve.

#9 Fish Nugget (Air Fryer)

Preparation Time: 10 minutes/Cooking Time: 6 Minutes/Serves: 2 Servings

Nutrition Per Serving: Carbohydrates: 6.4 grams/Fat: 7.6 grams/Protein: 22.3 grams/Fiber: 2.2 grams/Calories: 263

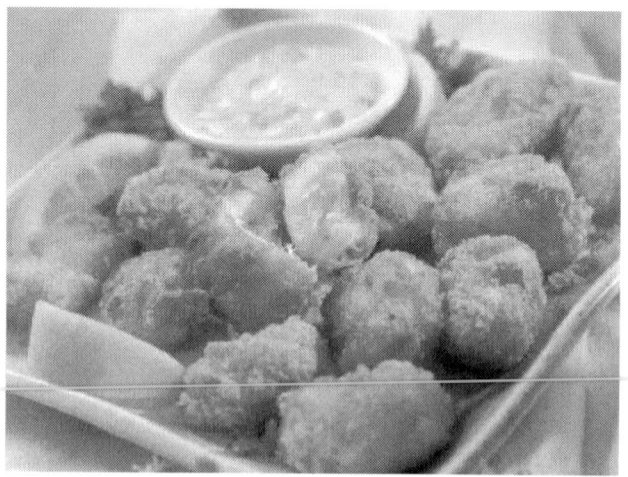

Ingredients

- 2 catfish fillets, skinless, each about 3 ounces
- ½ cup almond flour or all-purpose flour
- ½ teaspoon garlic powder
- 1 teaspoon salt
- ½ teaspoon ground black pepper
- ½ teaspoon smoked paprika
- 1 egg, at room temperature
- Non-stick cooking oil spray

Directions

1. Rinse the fish fillets, and pat dry with paper towels. Cut the fillets in bite-size pieces.
2. Crack the egg in a small bowl, and whisk until well blended.
3. Place flour in a shallow dish. Add garlic, salt, black pepper, and paprika and then stir until mixed.
4. Work on one fish piece at a time, dip into the egg and then coat in flour mixture.
5. Switch on the air fryer and grease the fryer's basket with oil. Insert it into the fryer and close the cover. Select the cooking temperature up to 425 degrees F and preheat.
6. Arrange the prepared fish nuggets in a single layer, and place into the fryer's basket. Spray with oil. Then fry for 10 minutes until crisp, turning halfway until thoroughly cooked.
7. When done, transfer the nuggets to a plate, and then serve.

Crab

#10 Steamed Crab Legs (Instant Pot)

Preparation Time: 10 minutes/Cooking Time: 3 Minutes/Serves: 2 Servings (1/2 pound per serving)

Nutrition Per Serving: Carbohydrates: 1.2 grams/Fat: 16 grams/Protein: 12.7 grams/Fiber: 0.3 grams/Calories: 199.4

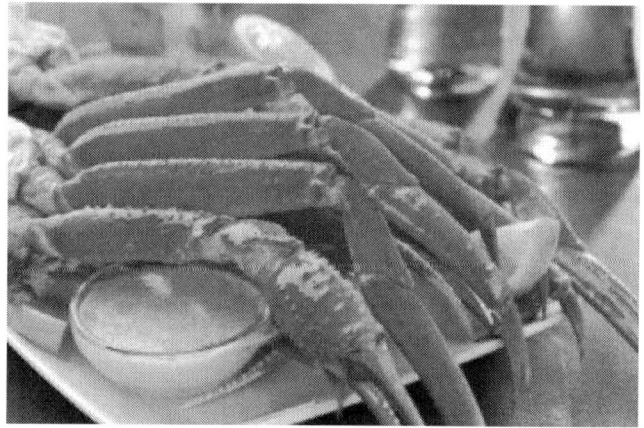

Ingredients

- 2 pounds king crab legs, frozen
- 1 lemon, juiced
- 1/3 cup butter, unsalted, melted
- 1 ½ cups water

Directions

1. Switch on the 4-quarts instant pot and pour water into the inner pot. Then insert the trivet stand or steamer basket in it.
2. Let the crab legs thaw for few minutes at room temperature. Place them on the trivet stand, and then close the cover of the instant pot securely.
8. Press the manual button and select the high-pressure setting. Set the cooking time to 3 minutes, and let it cook. The instant pot will take 5 to 10 minutes to build pressure, and then the cooking timer will start.
3. When the instant pot beeps, quickly release the pressure and open the instant pot carefully.
4. Transfer the steamed crab legs on a serving dish with tongs. Drizzle with lemon juice. Serve the crab legs with melted butter.

PESCATARIAN COOKBOOK FOR BEGINNERS

#11 Crab Bisque (Instant Pot)

Preparation Time: 10 minutes/Cooking Time: 8 Minutes/Serves: 4 Servings (1 bowl per serving)

Nutrition Per Serving: Carbohydrates: 10.7 grams/Fat: 35.1 grams/Protein: 13 grams/Fiber: 1.6 grams/Calories: 415

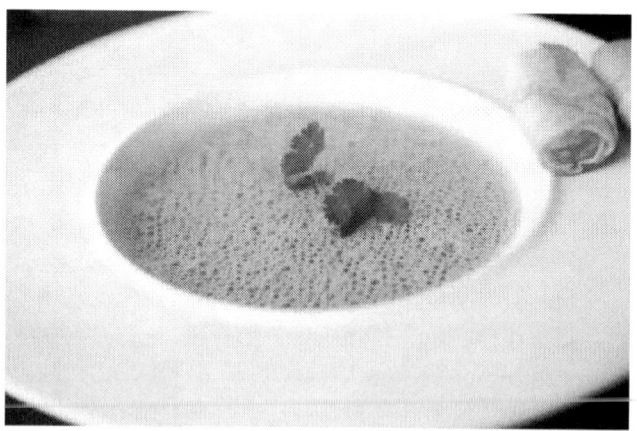

Ingredients

- 1-pound frozen crab meat, thawed
- ¼ cup chopped bell peppers
- 4 ounces white onion, peeled, thinly sliced
- 14 ounces crushed tomatoes
- 2 stalks of celery, chopped
- ½ teaspoon salt
- ½ teaspoon cayenne pepper
- 1 teaspoon Old Bay seasoning

- ½ teaspoon ground black pepper
- ¼ cup heavy whipping cream
- 4 tablespoons butter, unsalted, softened
- 3 cups chicken broth
- 8-ounces cream cheese, softened, full-fat

Directions

1. Switch on the 4-quarts instant pot. Press the sauté button and preheat.
2. Add butter, and let it melt. add the remaining ingredients. Stir until mixed, and then press the cancel button.
3. Close the instant pot's cover securely. Press the manual button and select the low-pressure setting. Set the cooking time to 3 minutes, and let it cook. The instant pot will take 5 to 10 minutes to build pressure, and then the cooking timer will start.
4. When the instant pot beeps, quickly release the pressure, and open the instant pot carefully.
5. Puree the mixture until it is smooth using an immersion blender and distribute evenly among 4 bowls.
6. Serve right away.

#12 Crab and Corn Chowder (Instant Pot)

Preparation Time: 10 minutes/Cooking Time: 10 Minutes/Serves: 4 Servings (1 bowl per serving)

Nutrition Per Serving: Carbohydrates: 30.3 grams/Fat: 15 grams/Protein: 11 grams/Fiber: 3 grams/Calories: 284

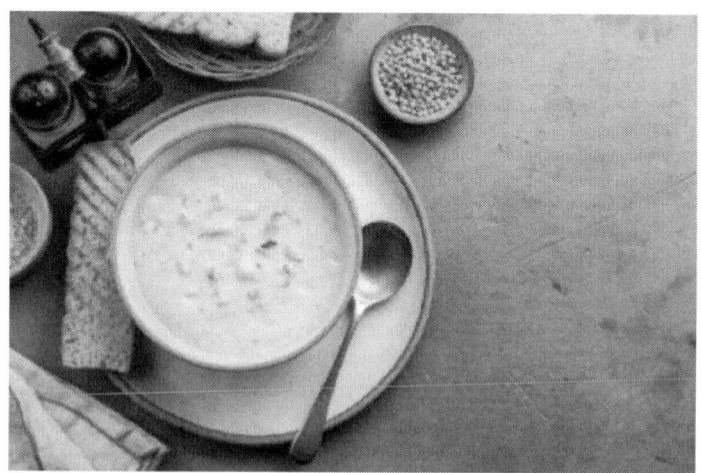

Ingredients

- 6 cups chopped cauliflower florets
- 1 cup chopped white onion
- 1 ½ cups sweet corn, frozen
- 1 cup chopped red bell pepper
- 8 ounces canned crab meat, picked through for shells
- ½ teaspoon salt

- ¼ teaspoon ground black pepper
- ¼ teaspoon cayenne pepper
- 2 teaspoons old bay seasoning
- 1 ½ cups milk, unsweetened
- 4 teaspoons butter, unsalted
- 1 ½ cups chicken broth

Directions

1. Switch on the 4-quarts instant pot. Press the sauté button and preheat.
2. Add butter, and let it melt. Add onion and bell pepper and stir until coated in butter. Then cook for 2 minutes until vegetable begins to soften.
3. Pour in the broth and stir until mixed. Press the cancel button, insert a steamer basket into the inner pot, and place chopped cauliflower florets.
4. Place the cover of the instant pot securely. Press the manual button and select the high-pressure setting. Set the cooking time to 3 minutes, and let it cook. The instant pot will take 5 to 10 minutes to build pressure, and then the cooking timer will start.
5. When the instant pot beeps, quickly release the pressure, and open the instant pot carefully.
6. Reserve 1 cup of steamed cauliflower florets and transfer the remaining florets into a blender. Add milk, and then blend until smooth.
7. Remove the steamer basket from the inner pot and add corn Press the manual button. Then cook for 2 to 3 minutes until thoroughly hot.

8. Add salt, old bay seasoning, cayenne pepper, and blended cauliflower. Then stir until mixed.
9. Add reserved cauliflower florets, stir until just mixed, and then place in 4 bowls.
10. Serve right away.

#13 Crab Cakes (Air Fryer)

Preparation Time: 5 minutes/Cooking Time: 10 Minutes/Serves: 4 Servings (1 cake per serving)

Nutrition Per Serving: Carbohydrates: 5 grams/Fat: 6 grams/Protein: 12 grams/Fiber: 1 grams/Calories: 123

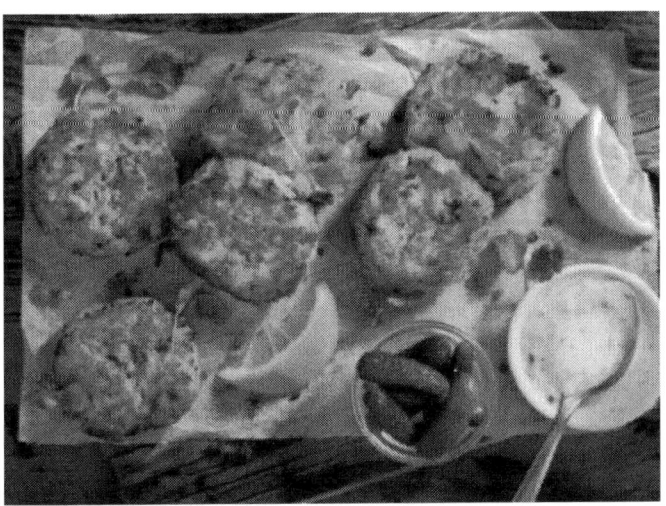

Ingredients

- 8-ounces lump crab
- ¼ cup chopped red bell pepper
- 2 green onion, chopped
- 1 teaspoon old bay seasoning
- 1 tablespoon Dijon mustard
- 2 tablespoons breadcrumbs
- 2 tablespoons mayonnaise
- Non-stick cooking oil spray

Directions

1. Switch on the air fryer, and line the fryer's basket with a foil. Grease it with oil and insert it into the fryer. Close the cover and select the cooking temperature up to 370 degrees F and preheat.
2. Meanwhile, place all the ingredients in a large bowl. Stir until well combined, and then shape the mixture into four evenly sized patties.
3. Arrange the prepared patties into the fryer's basket. Spray with oil and then fry for 10 minutes until golden brown, turning halfway.
4. Serve right away.

NATHALIE SEATON

Flatfish

#14 Crumbed Fish (Air Fryer)

Preparation Time: 5 minutes/Cooking Time: 24 Minutes/Serves: 4 Servings (1 fillet per serving)

Nutrition Per Serving: Carbohydrates: 22.5 grams/Fat: 17.7 grams/Protein: 27 grams/Fiber: 2.5 grams/Calories: 354.1

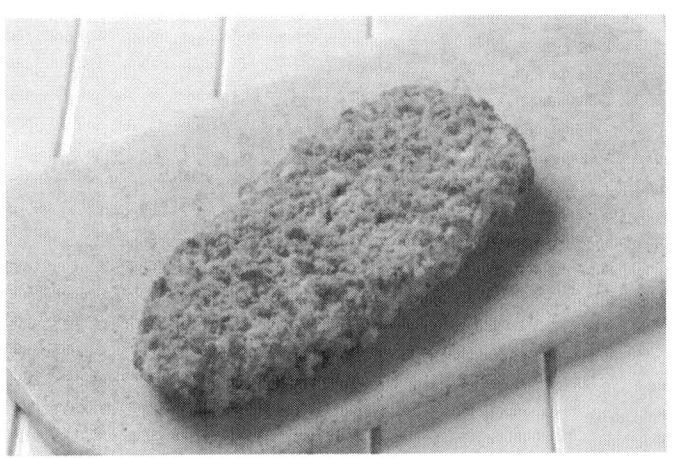

Ingredients

- 4 fillets of flounder, each about 4 to 6 ounces
- 1 cup breadcrumbs
- 1 egg, beaten
- 1 lemon, sliced
- ¼ cup olive oil

Directions

1. Switch on the air fryer and grease the its basket with oil. Insert it into the fryer and close the cover. Select the cooking temperature up to 350 degrees F and preheat.
2. Meanwhile, place the breadcrumbs in a shallow dish. Add oil, and then stir until crumbly mixture comes together.
3. Use another shallow dish and crack the egg. Then whisk until blended.
4. Work on 1 fillet at a time. Dip into the egg and then dredge in breadcrumbs until well coated.
5. Arrange the prepared fillets in a single layer, and place into the fryer's basket. Then fry for 12 minutes until golden brown, and fork-tender, turning halfway.
6. Serve the fillets with lemon slices.

#15 Zesty Ranch Fish Fillets (Air Fryer)

Preparation Time: 5 minutes/Cooking Time: 24 Minutes/Serves: 4 Servings (1 fillet per serving)

Nutrition Per Serving: Carbohydrates: 8 grams/Fat: 14 grams/Protein: 38 grams/Fiber: 2 grams/Calories: 315

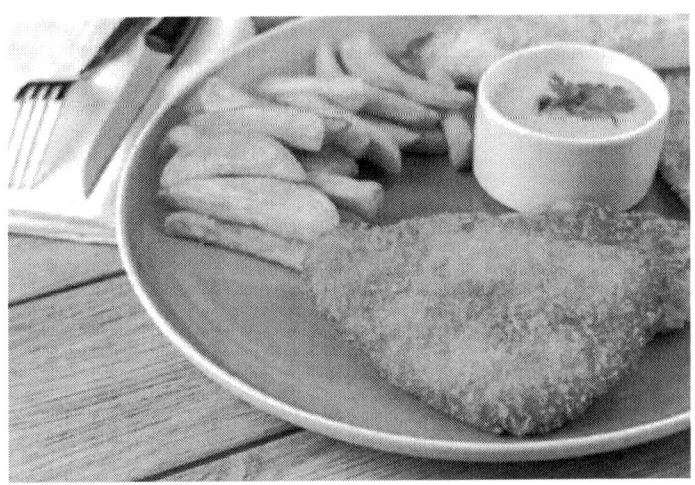

Ingredients

- 4 fillets of flounder, each about 4 to 6 ounces
- ¾ cup breadcrumbs
- 2 ½ tablespoons olive oil
- 30g packet of dry ranch-style dressing mix
- 2 eggs, beaten
- 1 lemon, cut into wedges

Directions

1. Switch on the air fryer and grease the frying basket with oil. Insert it into the fryer and close the cover. Select the cooking temperature up to 350 degrees F and preheat.
2. Meanwhile, get a shallow dish, place the breadcrumbs in it, then add ranch dressing mix and oil. Stir until crumbly mixture comes together.
3. Crack the egg in a shallow dish and then whisk until blended.
4. Work on 1 fillet at a time. Dip into the egg and then lightly coat in breadcrumbs mixture until well covered.
5. Arrange the prepared fillets in a single layer. Place into the fryer's basket, and fry for 12 minutes until golden brown and fork-tender, turning halfway.
6. Serve the fillets with lemon wedges.

#16 Parmesan Crusted White Fish (Air Fryer)

Preparation Time: 5 minutes/Cooking Time: 6 Minutes/Serves: 12 Servings (1 fillet per serving)

Nutrition Per Serving: Carbohydrates: 2 grams/Fat: 17 grams/Protein: 44 grams/Fiber: 1 grams/Calories: 338

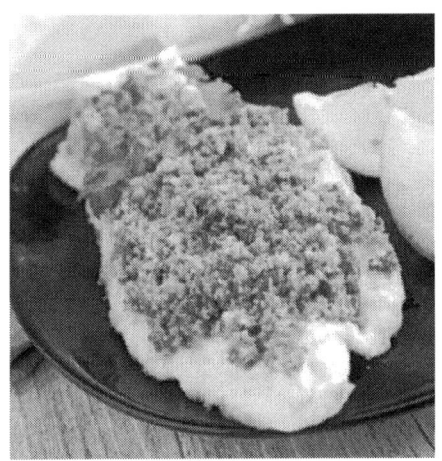

Ingredients

- 2 fillets of sole, each about 4 to 6 ounces
- ½ teaspoon onion powder
- ½ teaspoon salt
- ½ teaspoon garlic powder
- ¼ teaspoon ground black pepper
- ½ teaspoon smoked paprika
- 1 tablespoon fresh chopped parsley

- 1 tablespoon olive oil
- ½ cup grated parmesan cheese
- 1 lemon, cut into wedges
- Non-stick cooking oil spray

Directions

1. Switch on the air fryer, and line the frying basket with perforated parchment paper. Then grease it with oil.
2. Place the basket into the fryer and close the cover. Select the cooking temperature up to 350 degrees F and preheat.
3. Meanwhile, place grated parmesan cheese in a shallow dish.
4. Brush the fish fillets with oil, season with onion powder, salt, black pepper, garlic powder, and paprika. Press into the cheese until evenly coated.
5. Arrange the prepared fillets in a single layer. Place the fillets into the fryer's basket. Fry for 12 minutes until golden brown and fork-tender, turning halfway.
6. When done, transfer fish fillets onto a serving plate, sprinkle parsley on top, and then serve with lemon wedges.

#17 Grilled Flatfish with Herb Sauce (Griddle Pan)

Preparation Time: 15 minutes/Cooking Time: 15 Minutes/Serves: 4 Servings (1 piece per serving)

Nutrition Per Serving: Carbohydrates: 39.6 grams/Fat: 66.7 grams/Protein: 18.7 grams/Fiber: 4.5 grams/Calories: 835

Ingredients

- 1 whole sole or flounder, about 2 to 4 pounds, scaled
- 1 ½ teaspoon salt
- ½ teaspoon ground black pepper
- ½ teaspoon cayenne pepper
- Olive oil as needed
- For the Sauce:
- 2 cups chopped parsley
- 10 prunes, pits removed, chopped
- 1 cup chopped mint
- ½ teaspoon minced garlic
- ¼ cup raw pistachios
- ¼ cup chopped tarragon
- ½ teaspoon salt
- ¼ cup of soy sauce
- ¾ cup olive oil
- 2 tablespoons vinegar

Directions

1. Prepare the sauce and pour in a small skillet pan. Place it over medium-low heat and simmer.
2. Add pistachios and cook for 5 minutes until brown spots appear on them, stirring occasionally.
3. Let the pistachios cool completely, chop finely and transfer to a medium bowl.
4. Add remaining ingredients of the sauce. Stir until well blended. Then set aside.
5. Take a griddle pan, and grease it with oil. Place it over medium heat.
6. Cut the fish into pieces, about 2 or 4-inches wide, and pat dry with paper towels. Brush with oil, and season with salt, black pepper, and cayenne pepper.
7. Place the fish planks on the griddle pan and cook for 5 to 7 minutes until the skin can be easily removed.
8. Turn the fish and continue grilling for 3 to 5 minutes until the fish is thoroughly cooked.
9. When done, transfer grilled fish planks to a serving dish, spread sauce on top, and then serve.

#18 Pan-Fried Sole (Pan)

Preparation Time: 10 minutes/Cooking Time: 10 Minutes/Serves: 4 Servings (1 fillet per serving)

Nutrition Per Serving: Carbohydrates: 15 grams/Fat: 20 grams/Protein: 45 grams/Fiber: 1 grams/Calories: 424

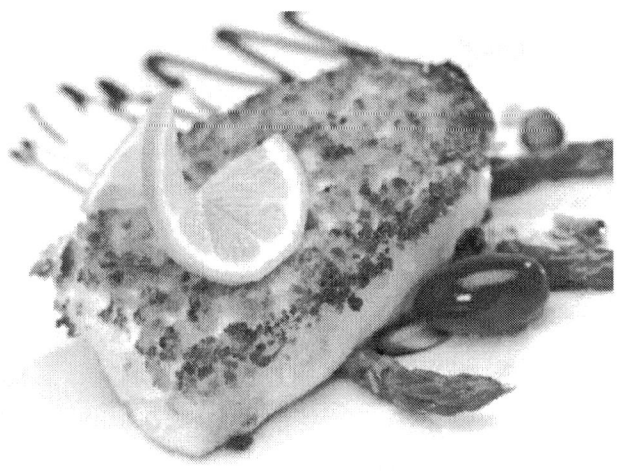

Ingredients

- 4 fillets of sole, each about 8-ounces
- ¼ teaspoon salt
- ½ teaspoon dried thyme
- ¼ teaspoon ground black pepper
- ¾ cup breadcrumbs
- 2 tablespoons olive oil
- 2 tablespoons butter, unsalted
- 2 eggs

Directions

1. Using a shallow dish, crack the eggs and then whisk until beaten.
2. Get another shallow dish, and place breadcrumbs in it. Add thyme, salt, and black pepper, and stir until mixed.
3. Work on one fillet at a time, and coat in breadcrumbs mixture. Dip into eggs, and then lightly coat into the breadcrumbs' mixture again until well covered.
4. Place a large skillet pan over medium-high heat. Add 1 tablespoon oil and 1 tablespoon butter, and heat until butter melts.
5. Add prepared fish fillets in a single layer, and then cook for 3 to 4 minutes per side until golden brown and fork-tender.
6. When done, transfer fillets to a serving dish. Add the remaining oil and butter and cook the remaining fillets in the same manner.
7. Serve right away.

Haddock

#19 Fish and Chips (Air Fryer)

Preparation Time: 5 minutes/Cooking Time: 24 Minutes/Serves: 4 Servings

Nutrition Per Serving: Carbohydrates: 37 grams/Fat: 5 grams/Protein: 28 grams/Fiber: 3 grams/Calories: 309

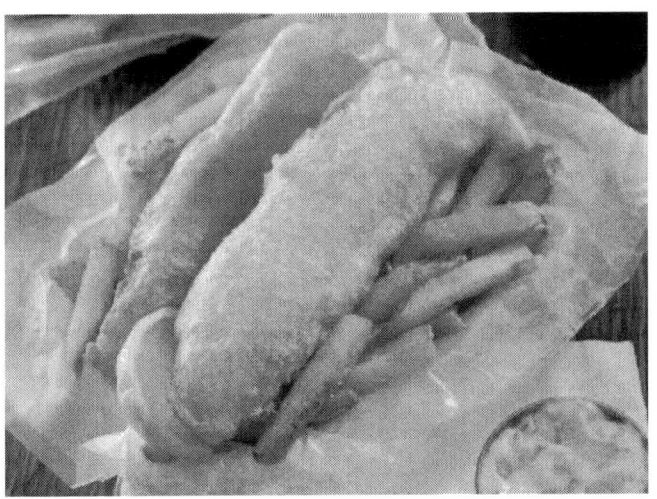

Ingredients

- 1-pound haddock fillets, cut into strips
- 2 cups panko breadcrumbs
- ½ cup all-purpose flour
- ¼ teaspoon salt
- ½ teaspoon garlic powder

- ¼ teaspoon ground black pepper
- 2 teaspoons paprika
- 1 egg
- 1 lemon, cut into wedges
- French fries as needed for serving

Directions

1. Switch on the air fryer and grease the fryer's basket with oil. Insert it into the fryer and close the cover. Select the cooking temperature up to 400 degrees F and preheat.
2. Meanwhile, place flour in a shallow dish. Add garlic powder, salt, and paprika, and then stir until mixed.
3. Use a separate shallow dish, crack the egg in it, and then whisk until beaten.
4. Place breadcrumbs in another shallow dish.
5. Work on one fish strip at a time, and dredge into the flour mixture. Dip into the egg and then lightly cover in breadcrumbs until coated.
6. Arrange the fish strips into the fryer's basket in a single layer, and spray with oil. Then fry for 12 to 14 minutes until golden brown and crisp, turning halfway.
7. Serve the fish strips with fries, favorite sauce, and lemon wedges.

#20 Haddock in Creamy Tomato Soup (Instant Pot)

Preparation Time: 5 minutes/Cooking Time: 20 Minutes/Serves: 4 Servings (1 bowl per serving)

Nutrition Per Serving: Carbohydrates: 28 grams/Fat: 20 grams/Protein: 24 grams/Fiber: 4 grams/Calories: 379

Ingredients

- 1-pound haddock fillets, wild-caught, frozen
- 2 cups chopped kale
- 1 medium white onion, peeled, sliced
- 2 cups whole peeled tomatoes, with juice
- 1 medium carrot, peeled, chopped
- ½ teaspoon minced garlic
- 1 large red potato, peeled, cubed
- 2 teaspoons sea salt
- 1/8 teaspoon crushed red pepper flakes
- 1 tablespoon fresh chopped basil
- ½ teaspoon ground black pepper
- 2 tablespoons fresh parsley, chopped
- 2 tablespoons butter, unsalted
- 2 cups chicken broth
- ½ cup heavy cream

Directions

1. Switch on the 4-quarts instant pot, and press the sauté button, and preheat.
2. Add butter, and let it melt. Add onion and garlic and stir until coated in butter. Cook for 3 minutes until the onion has softened.
3. Add tomatoes, potatoes, carrots, basil, and parsley. Pour-in chicken stock, stir until mixed, and then bring to a simmer.
4. Press the cancel button and insert a steamer basket. Season the fillets with salt, black pepper, and red pepper flakes. Stack the fillets on the steamer basket.
5. Close the cover of the instant pot securely. Press the manual button, then select the high-pressure setting. Cook for 6 minutes. The instant pot will take 5 to 10 minutes to build pressure, and then the cooking timer will start.
6. When the instant pot beeps, quickly release the pressure, and open the instant pot carefully.
7. Remove the fish along with the steamer rack from the instant pot. Then puree the broth mixture by using an immersion blender until smooth.
8. Press the keep warm function. Add fish, cream, and kale into the broth mixture. Stir until mixed and let it sit for 5 to 10 minutes until kale leaves wilts.
9. Scoop the haddock and broth mixture to evenly distribute in four bowls and then serve.

NATHALIE SEATON

#21 Haddock Pie (Instant Pot)

Preparation Time: 10 minutes/Cooking Time: 15 Minutes/Serves: 3 Servings

Nutrition Per Serving: Carbohydrates: 48.8 grams/Fat: 32.2 grams/Protein: 26.6 grams/Fiber: 7.2 grams/Calories: 591.7

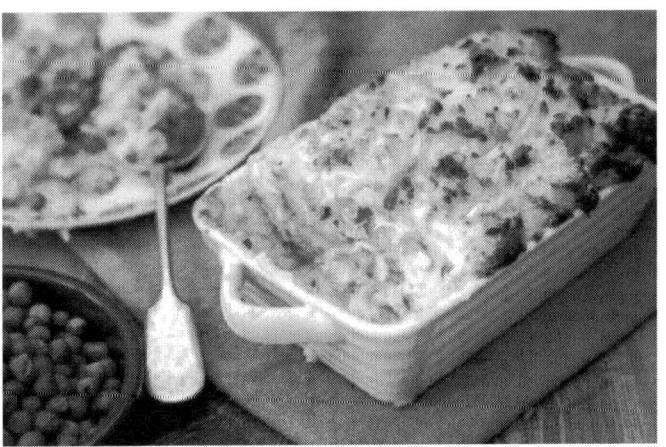

Ingredients

- 1-pound haddock, cut into bite-sizes pieces
- 10 ounces frozen corns
- 10 ounces of frozen peas
- 1 teaspoon salt
- ½ teaspoon ground black pepper
- ¼ cup breadcrumbs
- ½ cup cream cheese
- 2/3 cup milk, unsweetened
- ½ cup cheddar cheese shredded

Directions

1. Take a large bowl, pour in the milk, and then stir in cream cheese until well mixed.
2. Take another large bowl and place the haddock in it. Add corn and peas, and season with salt and black pepper. Then stir until combined.
3. Switch on the 4-quarts instant pot and scoop the haddock mixture in the inner pot and then add a layer with the prepared milk mixture.
4. Close the cover of the instant pot securely and press the manual button. Select the high-pressure setting, and then cook for 5 minutes. The instant pot will take 5 to 10 minutes to build pressure, by then, the cooking timer will start.
5. Meanwhile, switch on the oven, then set it up to 140 degrees F and preheat.
6. In a medium bowl, place breadcrumbs in it. Add cheese, and then stir until mixed.
7. When the instant pot beeps, let the pressure release naturally and then carefully open the instant pot.
8. Scoop the haddock mixture into a pie dish. Top with cheddar-breadcrumbs mixture, then bake for 10 minutes until the top turns golden brown.
9. When done, let the pie rest for 5 minutes and then serve.

#22 Panko Crusted Fried Haddock (Air Fryer)

Preparation Time: 5 minutes/Cooking Time: 24 Minutes/Serves: 4 Servings (1 fillet per serving)

Nutrition Per Serving: Carbohydrates: 33.7 grams/Fat: 21 grams/Protein: 43.7 grams/Fiber: 1.5 grams/Calories: 500

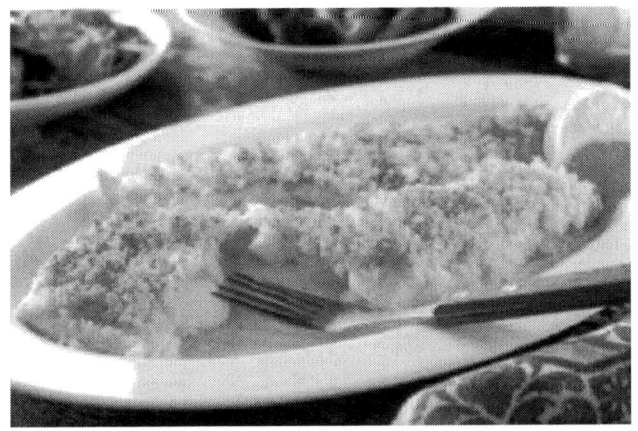

Ingredients

- 4 fillets of haddock fish, each about 5 ounces
- ½ cup all-purpose flour
- 1 teaspoon salt
- ½ teaspoon ground black pepper
- 6 tablespoons mayonnaise
- 2 eggs
- 3 cups panko breadcrumbs

Directions

1. Place salt and black pepper in a shallow dish. Add panko breadcrumbs, and then stir until mixed.
2. Use another shallow dish and place the flour in it.
3. Crack the eggs in another shallow dish, add mayonnaise and then whisk until blended.
4. Switch on the air fryer and grease the fryer's basket with oil. Insert it into the fryer and close the cover. Select the cooking temperature up to 350 degrees F and preheat.
5. Work on one fish fillet at a time, dredge into the flour mixture. Dip into the mayonnaise mixture, and then lightly coat into breadcrumbs mixture.
6. Arrange the prepared fish fillets in a single layer, and place into the fryer's basket. Spray with oil. Close the cover, and cook for 12 minutes until golden brown, and crisp, turning halfway through and spraying with oil.
7. Serve right away.

#23 Lemon Pepper Haddock (Air Fryer)

Preparation Time: 10 minutes/Cooking Time: 12 Minutes/Serves: 1 Serving (1 fillet per serving)

Nutrition Per Serving: Carbohydrates: 47 grams/Fat: 1.3 grams/Protein: 51.1 grams/Fiber: 3 grams/Calories: 409

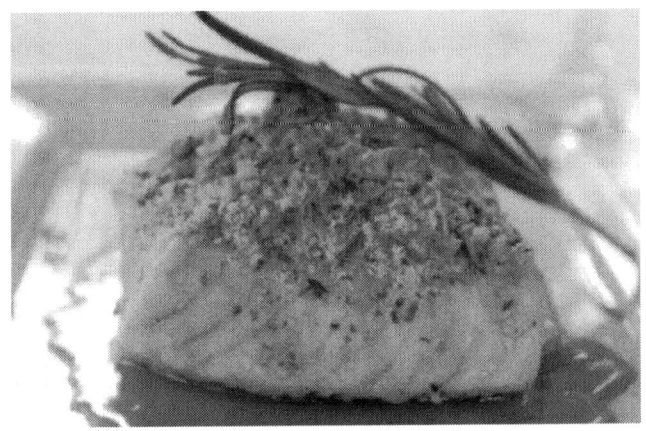

Ingredients

- 1 fillet of haddock, about 8 ounces
- 1/3 cup panko breadcrumbs
- ¼ cup all-purpose flour
- 2 teaspoons lemon pepper seasoning
- 2 egg whites
- 2 slices of lemon
- 2 tablespoons chopped parsley

Directions

1. Switch on the air fryer and grease the fryer's basket with oil. Insert it into the fryer and close the cover. Select the cooking temperature up to 350 degrees F and preheat.
2. Get a shallow dish, and place flour in it.
3. Use another shallow dish, and place egg whites. Then whisk until blended.
4. Add breadcrumbs, and lemon pepper seasoning in a shallow dish, then stir until mixed.
5. First, lightly coat the fish into the flour. Dip into the egg, and then coat the fish into the breadcrumbs 'mixture, pressing into the fish.
8. Place the prepared fish into the fryer's basket, and spray with oil. Close the cover, and then cook for 12 minutes until golden brown and crisp, turning halfway, and spraying with oil.
6. When done, garnish with parsley and serve the fish with lemon slices.

Herring

#24 Oat-Crusted Fried Herring (Air Fryer)

Preparation Time: 15 minutes/Cooking Time: 12 Minutes/Serves: 2 Servings

Nutrition Per Serving: Carbohydrates: 47 grams/Fat: 19 grams/Protein: 33 grams/Fiber: 9 grams/Calories: 488

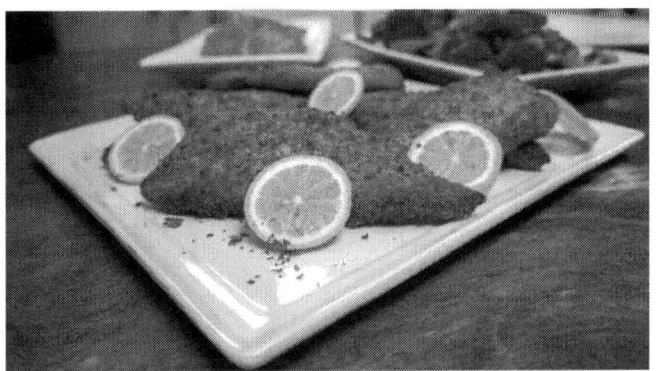

Ingredients

- ½ pound herring fillets
- 1 ½ cups oats
- 1 teaspoon salt
- ½ cup Dijon mustard
- ½ cup cream
- Non-stick cooking oil spray

Directions

1. Rinse the fish fillet, and pat dry with paper towels. Then, season well with salt.
2. Place cream and mustard in a shallow dish, and whisk until well mixed.
3. Add seasoned herring in it and toss until coated. Then, let it stand at room temperature for 10 minutes.
4. Meanwhile, switch on the air fryer, and grease the fryer's basket with oil. Insert it into the fryer and close the cover. Select the cooking temperature up to 400 degrees F and preheat.
5. Place the oats in a blender or food processor. Start the blender until mixture looks like flour, and then place it into a shallow dish.
6. Dredge fillets into the oat mixture until well coated, and then arrange in a single layer, then place into the fryer's basket.
7. Spray oil over the fillets and close the cover. Cook for 12 minutes until golden brown and crisp, turning halfway and spraying with oil.
8. Serve right away.

#25 Caribbean Fried Smoked Herring (Pan)

Preparation Time: 10 minutes/Cooking Time: 15 Minutes/Serves: 3 Servings

Nutrition Per Serving: Carbohydrates: 21 grams/Fat: 25 grams/Protein: 12 grams/Fiber: 3 grams/Calories: 348

Ingredients

- 8 ounces smoked herring fillets
- ½ cup diced white onions
- 1 hot pepper, minced
- ½ cup diced tomatoes
- 2 green onions, thinly sliced, white and green parts separated
- ½ teaspoon minced garlic
- 2 tablespoons olive oil
- 1 tablespoon minced thyme
- ½ tablespoon lemon juice
- Water as needed

Directions

1. Use a medium saucepan, place it over medium-high heat. Add herring fillets, and then cover with water.
2. Bring to a boil. Let the fish boil for 5 minutes, then drain the water completely and set aside until needed.

3. Let the fish cool slightly, and then chop into small pieces, and set aside.
4. Get a large skillet pan, place it over medium heat, and add oil.
5. Add onion, toss until coated in oil. Then cook for 5 minutes until onions have turned tender.
6. Add garlic, tomatoes, thyme, and hot pepper. Stir until mixed, and then continue cooking for 1 minute.
7. Add the drained herring into the pan and toss until well mixed. Cook for 5 minutes, and then stir in green onions, and lemon juice.
8. Remove the pan from heat and serve immediately.

#26 Fried Herring (Air Fryer)

Preparation Time: 10 minutes/Cooking Time: 20 Minutes/Serves: 4 Servings (1 fish per serving)

Nutrition Per Serving: Carbohydrates: 10.9 grams/Fat: 9.4 grams/Protein: 37 grams/Fiber: 0.9 grams/Calories: 276

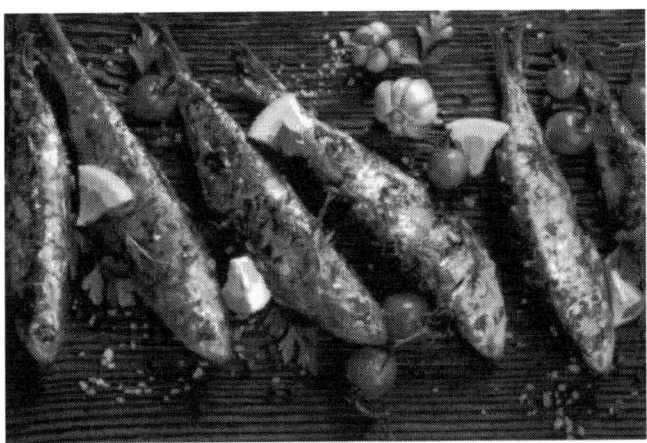

Ingredients

- 5 herrings, scaled, gutted, cleaned, rinsed
- 5 tablespoons pastry flour or all-purpose flour
- 2 teaspoons salt
- 2 teaspoons ground black pepper
- ½ cup chopped parsley
- 1 lemon, cut into wedges
- Non-stick cooking oil spray

Directions

1. Switch on the air fryer and grease the fryer's basket with oil. Insert it into the fryer and close the cover. Select the cooking temperature up to 400 degrees F and preheat.
2. Prepare the herring. Remove the scales, its insides, and then rinse well.
3. Season the herring with salt, and black pepper, then coat it with flour.
4. Arrange the prepared herring in a single layer into the fryer' basket, and spray with oil. Close the cover, and then cook for 10 minutes until golden brown and crisp, turning halfway, and spraying with oil.
5. When done, transfer fried herring to a plate. Garnish with parsley, and then serve with lemon wedges.

NATHALIE SEATON

#27 Smoked Salmon and Herring on Toasted Baguette (Oven)

Preparation Time: 10 minutes/Cooking Time: 10 Minutes/Serves: 6 Servings (2 toasts per serving)

Nutrition Per Serving: Carbohydrates: 15.1 grams/Fat: 7.9 grams/Protein: 11.5 grams/Fiber: 0.7 grams/Calories: 178

Ingredients

- 7 ounces smoked salmon
- 1 teaspoon salt
- 3 ounces canned herring fillets, chopped
- ½ teaspoon dried thyme
- ½ teaspoon dried parsley
- ½ teaspoon ground black pepper
- ½ teaspoon dried rosemary
- 1 tablespoon lemon zest
- 1 tablespoon chopped fresh dill
- 2 tablespoons lemon juice
- 1 ciabatta baguette
- 2 tablespoons olive oil

Directions

1. Switch on the oven and set it up to 400 degrees F and preheat.

2. Meanwhile, cut the baguette in half (lengthwise), and brush the inside with oil. Then sprinkle it with salt.
3. Place the cut baguettes into the oven. Bake for 5 minutes, or more until slightly toasted.
4. When done, sprinkle thyme, parsley, black pepper, and rosemary on the baguettes. Cut each baguette into six slices.
5. Top each baguette slice with herring and salmon. Sprinkle lemon zest and dill on top, and then drizzle with lemon juice.
6. Serve right away.

NATHALIE SEATON

Lobster

#28 Lobster Tails (Instant Pot)

Preparation Time: 10 minutes/Cooking Time: 1 Minutes/Serves: 2 Servings (1 lobster tail per serving)

Nutrition Per Serving: Carbohydrates: 0.7 grams/Fat: 24 grams/Protein: 21 grams/Fiber: 0 grams/Calories: 301

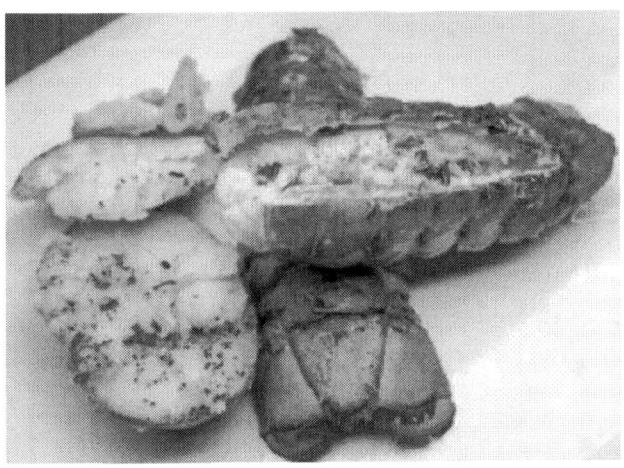

Ingredients

- 2 lobster tails
- 1 teaspoon of sea salt
- 1 teaspoon garlic powder
- ½ teaspoon ground white pepper
- 1 teaspoon smoked paprika

- 1 ½ tablespoon butter, unsalted, divided
- 1 cup of water
- ¼ cup melted butter, unsalted

Directions

1. Switch on the 4-quarts instant pot and fill the inner pot with water. Insert a trivet stand.
2. Place a lobster tail on a baking sheet, and then cut the top of the tail shell down to its tip with kitchen scissors.
3. Remove any grit or vein from the lobster tail. Pull the shell down so that meat looks on top of crab shell. Slide a lemon wedge between the lobster's tail and meat. Do the same with the other lobster tail.
4. Place salt in a small bowl. Add garlic powder, white pepper, and paprika. Stir until well mixed, and then sprinkle mixture on the meat.
5. Top the meat with small pieces of butter and arrange the crabs' tails on the trivet stand. Close the cover of the instant pot securely.
9. Press the manual button, sand elect the high-pressure setting. Cook for 1 minute. The instant pot will take 5 to 10 minutes to build pressure, and then the cooking timer will start.
6. When the instant pot beeps, quickly release the pressure, and open the instant pot. Let the lobster tail rest in the instant pot for 10 minutes.
7. Place the lobster tail to a serving dish and then serve with melted butter.

NATHALIE SEATON

#29 Lobster Risotto (Instant Pot)

Preparation Time: 5 minutes/Cooking Time: 25 Minutes/Serves: 2 Servings (1 bowl per serving)

Nutrition Per Serving: Carbohydrates: 43 grams/Fat: 8 grams/Protein: 21 grams/Fiber: 0 grams/Calories: 339

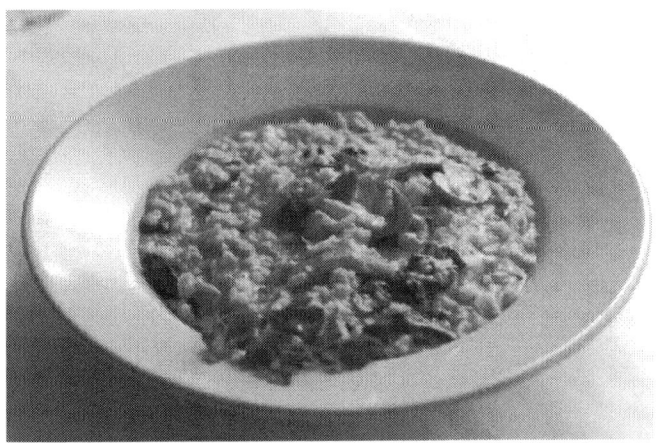

Ingredients

- 1 cup Arborio rice, rinsed
- 2 lobster tails, each about 4 ounces
- 1 large shallot, peeled, minced
- 1 ½ teaspoon minced garlic
- 1 leek, sliced
- ¾ teaspoon salt
- 1/3 teaspoon ground black pepper
- 1 tablespoon chopped thyme leaves

- 1 tablespoon butter, unsalted
- 1 tablespoon olive oil
- ½ cup brandy
- 3 tablespoon mascarpone cheese
- 2 cups fish stock
- 1 tablespoon chopped thyme leaves

Directions

1. Fill a large pot with a half full salted water. Place it over medium-high heat and bring to a boil.
2. Add lobster tails, boil for 7 minutes, or more until the tails curl and turn bright red in color. Then, drain the remaining water.
3. Let the lobster tails cool for 10 minutes, cut them open by cutting lengthwise along the back of the shell. Use a kitchen shear, and then chop the lobsters' meat. Set aside until needed.
4. Switch on the 4-quarts instant pot and press the sauté button.
5. Add butter and oil into the inner pot and let the butter melts. Add shallots and leeks, and then cook for 2 minutes until vegetables begin to soften.
6. Add garlic and stir until well mixed. Cook for 1 minute, then add rice. Stir until well combined.
7. Pour brandy into the inner pot and bring it to a simmer. Pour in the fish stock and stir until well blended. Press the cancel button.

10. Close the cover of the instant pot securely. Press the manual button and select the high-pressure setting. Cook for 6 minutes. The instant pot will take 5 to 10 minutes to build pressure, and then the cooking timer will start.
8. When the instant pot beeps, quickly release the pressure, and then open the instant pot carefully.
9. Add salt, black pepper, and cheese into the risotto. Stir until cheese melts, and then place evenly in two bowls.
10. Top the risotto with lobsters' meat, and garnish with thyme, then serve.

#30 Lobster and Bacon Chowder (Instant Pot)

Preparation Time: 5 minutes/Cooking Time: 25 Minutes/Serves: 6 Servings (1 bowl per serving)

Nutrition Per Serving: Carbohydrates: 20.1 grams/Fat: 13.1 grams/Protein: 11.3 grams/Fiber: 2 grams/Calories: 236.5

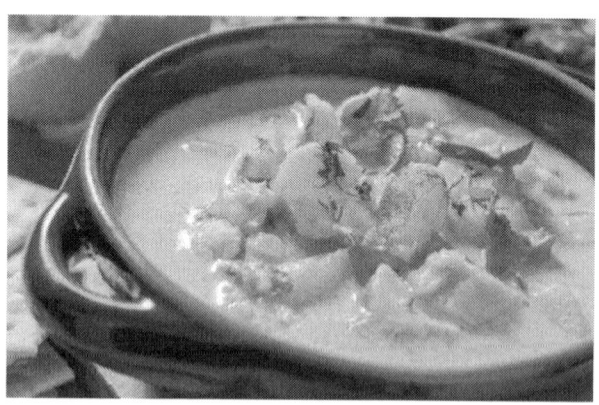

Ingredients

- 2 cups canned lobster meat
- 2 leeks, thinly sliced
- 3 cups frozen corn kernels
- 2 stalks of celery, diced
- 4 bacon slices, diced
- 2 medium red potatoes, unpeeled, diced
- 1 teaspoon salt
- 1 tablespoon corn starch

- ½ teaspoon ground black pepper
- 1 cup heavy cream
- 4 cups lobster stock or chicken broth
- 2 tablespoons chopped chives

Directions

1. Switch on the 4-quarts instant pot and press the sauté button. Preheat until hot.
2. Add bacon slices and cook for 5 minutes until crisp. Transfer bacon to a plate, and reserve 1 tablespoon of bacon fat from the inner pot.
3. Add leeks, and celery into the inner pot. Cook for 3 minutes until vegetables become soft and press the cancel button.
4. Return cooked bacon into the inner pot and add corn and potatoes. Pour in the stock and stir until well combined.
5. Close the cover of the instant pot securely. Press the manual button and select the high-pressure setting. Cook for 7 minutes. The instant pot will take 5 to 10 minutes to build pressure, and then the cooking timer will start.
6. Meanwhile, using a small bowl, add cream, and whisk in cornstarch until well combined.
7. When the instant pot beeps, quickly release pressure, and then carefully open the instant pot.
8. Press the sauté button and add the cream mixture. Stir for 1 minute and bring the chowder to a simmer. Cook for 1 to 2 minutes until chowder has thickened.

9. Add lobster meat and stir until mixed. Simmer for 3 to 4 minutes until thoroughly hot, and then press the cancel button.
10. Season the chowder with salt and black pepper. Garnish with chives, and then serve.

#31 Grilled Lobster with Garlic-Parsley Butter (Griddle Pan)

Preparation Time: 10 minutes/Cooking Time: 10 Minutes/Serves: 2 Servings (1 lobster half per serving)

Nutrition Per Serving: Carbohydrates: 1.7 grams/Fat: 72.4 grams/Protein: 14.1 grams/Fiber: 0 grams/Calories: 708

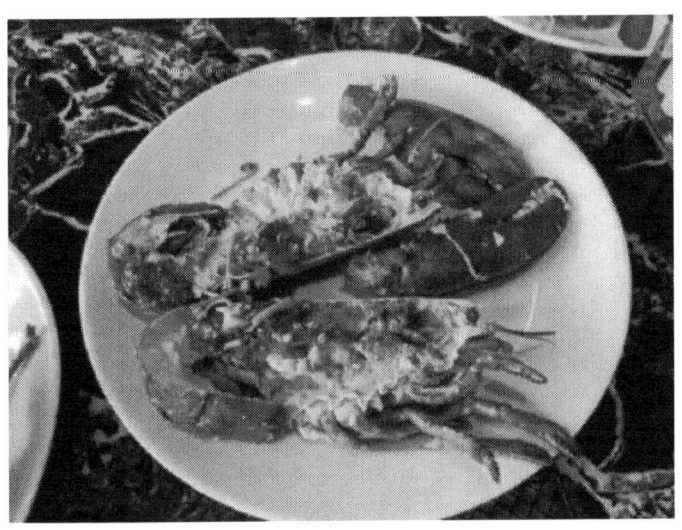

Ingredients

- 1 lobster, about 1 ½ pound
- 2 teaspoons minced garlic
- 1 lemon, zested
- 1 teaspoon salt
- 1 ½ teaspoon crushed red chili flakes

- ½ teaspoon ground black pepper
- 2 tablespoons chopped parsley
- ¼ cup olive oil
- 8 tablespoons butter, unsalted, softened

Directions

1. Using a medium bowl, place parsley, garlic, and butter in it. Add salt, black pepper, lemon zest, parsley, and red chili flakes. Then stir until combined, set aside until needed.
2. Set up the grill and set it to a high-heat setting. Preheat. A large griddle pan can also be used.
3. Meanwhile, prepare the lobster, split it in half lengthwise from head to tail by using a cleaver. Break off its claws, and then discard its green-yellow tomalley.
4. Place lobster halves on a large baking sheet, shell-side down along with claws. Drizzle with oil, and then season with salt, and black pepper.
5. Place the prepared lobster halves flesh-side-down and claws on the grill, and then cook for 3 minutes until slightly charred.
6. Carefully turn the lobster meat and spread the prepared garlic-parsley mixture over it and continue grilling for 5 minutes.
7. Serve right away.

NATHALIE SEATON

Mackerel

#32 Marinated Mackerel (Griddle Pan)

Preparation Time: 25 minutes /Cooking Time: 12 Minutes/Serves: 4 Servings (1 fillet)

Nutrition Per Serving: Carbohydrates: 0.8 grams/Fat: 26.7 grams/Protein: 20.3 grams/Fiber: 0.1 grams/Calories: 326

Ingredients

- 4 fillets of mackerel, with skin, each about 4 to 6 ounces
- 1 teaspoon salt
- 1 teaspoon ground black pepper
- Non-stick cooking oil spray
  For the Marinade:
- ½ tablespoon grated ginger
- ½ tablespoon minced garlic
- 3 tablespoons soy sauce
- 2 tablespoons olive oil
- 1 lemon, juiced

Directions

1. Using a large bowl, place all the ingredients to be marinated. Stir until well blended.
2. Add mackerel fillets and toss until coated. Cover the bowl, and then let the fish marinate for a minimum of 20 minutes.
3. Get a griddle pan. Grease it with oil and place over medium-high heat.
4. Arrange the marinated fish fillets on the griddle pan (skin-side up) and cook for 5 minutes.
5. Turn the fish fillets, and drizzle with the remaining marinade. Season with salt, and black pepper. Continue cooking for 5 to 7 minutes until fillets have thoroughly cooked.
6. Serve right away or serve with boiled rice.

#33 Mackerel Fish Fry (Air Fryer)

Preparation Time: 25 minutes /Cooking Time: 12 Minutes/Serves: 5 Servings (1 fish per serving)

Nutrition Per Serving: Carbohydrates: 1.3 grams/Fat: 42.8 grams/Protein: 30.8 grams/Fiber: 0.02 grams/Calories: 515

Ingredients

- 5 whole mackerel fish, gutted, cleaned
- 1 lemon, cut into wedges
- Non-stick cooking oil spray
  For the Marinade:
- 1 teaspoon minced garlic
- ½ teaspoon grated ginger
- 3 sprigs of curry leaves, chopped
- 1 tablespoon red chili powder
- 1 teaspoon salt
- 1 teaspoon red chili flakes
- ½ teaspoon turmeric powder
- ½ teaspoon vinegar
- 3 tablespoons olive oil, melted

Directions

1. Prepare the fish. Remove its inside, rinse well until cleaned, and pat dry. Make 3 to 4 small cuts on each fish.
2. Using a small bowl, place all the ingredients to be marinated, and stir until well combined.
3. Brush the marinade on all sides of each fish. Make sure it goes into the cut and the fish is evenly seasoned. Marinate the fish for a minimum of 20 minutes in the refrigerator.
4. When ready to cook, switch on the air fryer, and grease its frying basket with oil. Insert it into the fryer and close the cover. Select the cooking temperature up to 400 degrees F and preheat.
5. Arrange the marinated fish in a single layer, and place in the fryer's basket. Set the frying time to 12 minutes, and then let it cook until fork tender.
6. When done, transfer the fish to a plate and then serve with lemon wedges.

NATHALIE SEATON

#34 Fried Crumbed Mackerel (Air Fryer)

Preparation Time: 10 minutes/Cooking Time: 12 Minutes/Serves: 4 Servings (1 fish per serving)

Nutrition Per Serving: Carbohydrates: 27.5 grams/Fat: 45.8 grams/Protein: 43 grams/Fiber: 1.4 grams/Calories: 690

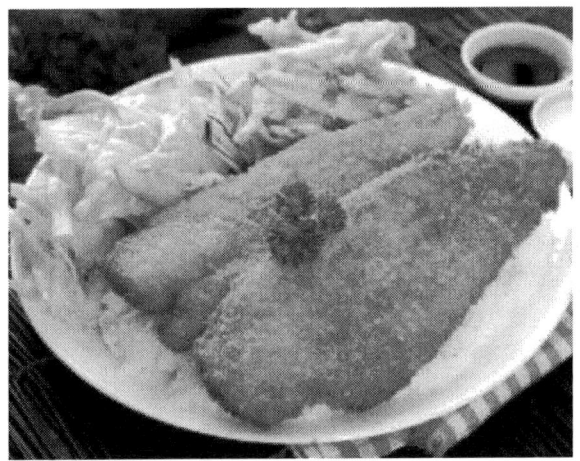

Ingredients

- 4 mackerel fish, gutted, cleaned
- ¾ cup breadcrumbs
- ½ cup tempura flour
- ½ teaspoon garlic powder
- ½ teaspoon salt
- ½ cup of water
- Non-stick cooking oil spray

Directions

1. Prepare the mackerel fish. Remove its head, tail, and insides. Rinse well until clean, and then pat dry.
2. Cut the fish into bite-size pieces. Place in a large bowl, season with salt and garlic powder Then toss until coated.
3. Take a separate bowl, and place tempura flour in it. Whisk in water until smooth batter comes together, and let it rest for 15 minutes.
4. Spread breadcrumbs in a shallow dish.
5. Switch on the air fryer and grease its frying basket with oil. Insert it into the fryer and close the cover. Select the cooking temperature up to 400 degrees F and preheat.
6. Work on one fish piece at a time. Dip the fish into the tempura flour mixture, and then lightly coat in breadcrumbs until all side are covered.
7. Then arrange the prepared fish pieces in a single layer. Place them in the fryer's basket. Set the frying time to 12 minutes, and let it cook until crispy, turning halfway and spraying with oil.
8. When done, transfer fried mackerel to a plate, and then serve with chili sauce.

NATHALIE SEATON

#35 Fried Mackerel with Ginger Sauce (Pan)

Preparation Time: 20 minutes/Cooking Time: 12 Minutes/Serves: 2 Servings (1 fillet per serving)

Nutrition Per Serving: Carbohydrates: 6 grams/Fat: 33.4 grams/Protein: 20.3 grams/Fiber: 0.2 grams/Calories: 406

Ingredients

- 2 fillets of Mackerel, skin on, each about 4 to 6 ounces
- 1 teaspoon salt
- 2 tablespoons olive oil
  For the Sauce:
- 2 teaspoons chopped garlic
- ¼ teaspoon sugar
- 3 teaspoons chopped ginger
- 1 tablespoon corn starch
- 1 teaspoon oyster sauce
- ½ cup and 2 tablespoons water, divided
- 1 teaspoon soy sauce

Directions

1. Rinse the fillets, and pat dry. Place them on a cutting board (skin-side up). Make a criss-cross pattern on the flesh.
2. Cut each fillet in half, season with salt until coated on all sides. Let the fillets rest for 15 minutes.
3. Using a large frying pan, place it over medium heat and add oil.
4. Add fish fillet, and cook for 3 to 4 minutes per side, or until fork tender. Then transfer to a plate.
5. Prepare the sauce by adding ginger and garlic. Cook for 1 minute until fragrant.
6. Pour in ½ cup water, soy sauce, sugar, and oyster sauce, and then stir until well mixed.
7. Get a small bowl, add cornstarch, and stir in remaining water until smooth. Place the mixture in a frying pan.
8. Cook the sauce for 2 to 3 minutes until thickened to the desired level, and then pour into a serving bowl.
9. Serve the sauce with fish fillets.

#36 Lemon Garlic Mackerel (Griddle Pan)

Preparation Time: 15 minutes/Cooking Time: 10 Minutes/Serves: 4 Servings (1 fillet per serving)

Nutrition Per Serving: Carbohydrates: 1 grams/Fat: 13.9 grams/Protein: 18.7 grams/Fiber: 0.1 grams/Calories: 208.7

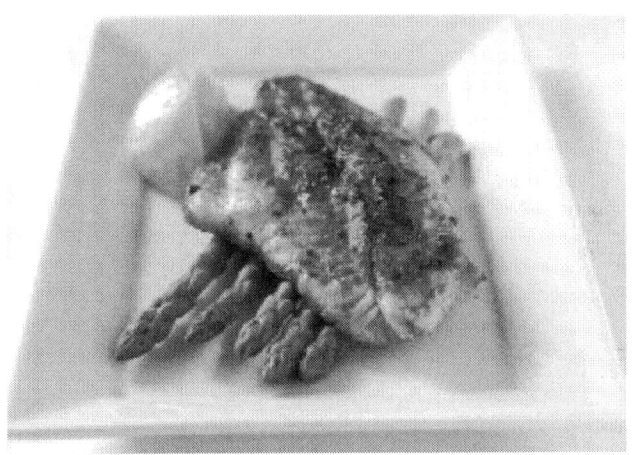

Ingredients

- 4 fillets of mackerel, skin on
- 1 teaspoon minced garlic
- ½ teaspoon salt
- ½ teaspoon ground black pepper
- ½ of lemon, juiced
- Non-stick cooking oil spray

Directions

1. Line the baking tray with foil. Place the fillet on it, and sprinkle with salt. Let it rest for 10 minutes.
2. Meanwhile, using a griddle pan, grease it with oil. Place it over medium-high heat.
3. Place garlic in a small bowl, then, add black pepper and lemon juice. Stir until mixed.
4. After 10 minutes, pour the lemon mixture over the mackerel fillets, and then toss until coated.
5. Arrange the fish fillets on the griddle pan. Cook for 5 minutes per side until fork-tender.
6. Serve immediately.

#37 Teriyaki Mackerel (Air Fryer)

Preparation Time: 5 minutes/Cooking Time: 25 Minutes/Serves: 5 Servings (1/2-pound fillets per serving)

Nutrition Per Serving: Carbohydrates: 24 grams/Fat: 29.7 grams/Protein: 28.6 grams/Fiber: 0.8 grams/Calories: 478

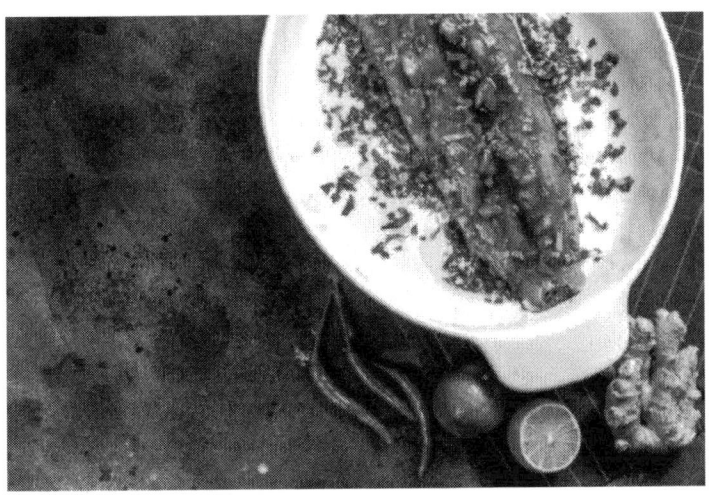

Ingredients

- 1½ lbs mackerel fillets, skin on
- 2 green onions, sliced
- Non-stick cooking oil spray
  For the Teriyaki sauce:
- ½ teaspoon minced garlic
- ½ cup maple syrup or honey

- 2 teaspoons chopped ginger
- 1 cup of soy sauce
- 1 lemon, zested
- 1 cup of rice wine

Directions

1. Place a medium saucepan over medium heat, then add all the ingredients for the sauce. Stir until well combined.
2. Bring the sauce to a boil, and switch heat to medium-low level. Let it simmer for 15 to 20 minutes until reduced by half. Uncover the pan and when done, strain the sauce.
3. Switch on the air fryer and grease its frying basket with oil. Insert it into the fryer and close the cover. Select the cooking temperature up to 400 degrees F and preheat.
4. Brush the fish fillets with the prepared teriyaki sauce. Arrange the fillets into the fryer basket (skin-side down). Set the frying time to 5 minutes, and then let it cook.
5. After 5 minutes, turn the fillets, and brush with the teriyaki sauce. Continue frying for 5 minutes until fillets have turned fork tender.
6. When done, transfer fish fillets to a plate, and drizzle with remaining teriyaki sauce. Sprinkle with green onions, and then serve.

#38 Honey Soy Mackerel (Air Fryer)

Preparation Time: 30 minutes /Cooking Time: 10 Minutes/Serves: 4 Servings (1 fillet per serving)

Nutrition Per Serving: Carbohydrates: 4.2 grams/Fat: 46.8 grams/Protein: 30.8 grams/Fiber: 0.7 grams/Calories: 562

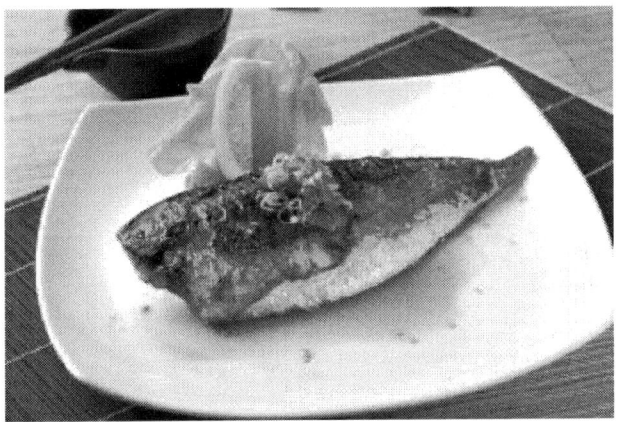

Ingredients

- 4 whole mackerel, gutted, cleaned
  For the Marinade:
- 1 red chili, chopped
- 1 lime, juiced, zested
- 1 teaspoon minced garlic
- 1 teaspoon honey
- 2 tablespoons soy sauce
- 4 tablespoons olive oil
- 1 tablespoon sesame oil

Directions

1. Place all the ingredients for the marinade in a large bowl, and whisk until combined.
2. Prepare the mackerel. Remove its head, tail, and insides. Rinse well until clean, and pat dry.
3. Add the fish into the prepared marinade and toss until well coated. Cover the bowl with its lid, and then let the fish marinate for a minimum of 20 minutes at room temperature.
4. Switch on the air fryer. Grease its frying basket with oil and insert it into the fryer. Close the cover and select the cooking temperature up to 400 degrees F and preheat.
5. Arrange the marinated fish in a single layer, and place in the fryer's basket. Set the frying time to 10 minutes, and let it cook until fork-tender, turning halfway and spraying with oil.
6. Serve right away.

Mullet

#39 Blackened Mullet (Air Fryer)

Preparation Time: 10 minutes/Cooking Time: 10 Minutes/Serves: 6 Servings (1/2 pound per serving)

Nutrition Per Serving: Carbohydrates: 1.2 grams/Fat: 22.4 grams/Protein: 60.4 grams/Fiber: 0.2 grams/Calories: 449

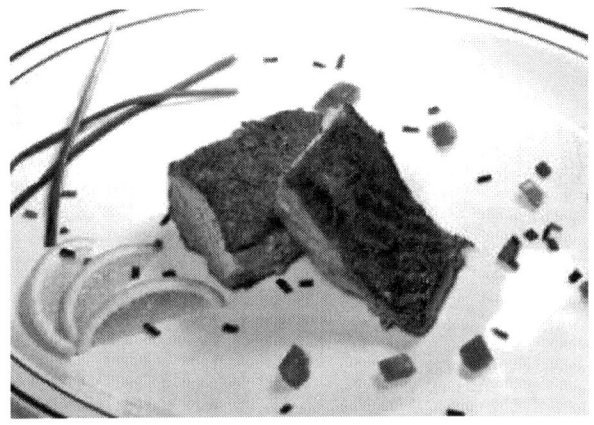

Ingredients

- 3 pounds mullet fillets, skinless
- ¼ cup butter, unsalted, melted
- Non-stick cooking oil spray
  The Spice Mix:
- ½ tablespoon garlic powder

- ½ tablespoon onion powder
- ½ teaspoon ground black pepper
- ½ teaspoon mustard powder
- ½ teaspoon cayenne pepper
- ¾ teaspoon salt
- ½ teaspoon dried thyme
- ½ tablespoon sweet paprika

Directions

1. Using a small bowl, place all the ingredients for the spice mix, and then stir until well blended.
2. Switch on the air fryer and grease its frying basket with oil. Insert it into the fryer and close the cover. Select the cooking temperature up to 400 degrees F and preheat.
3. Meanwhile, brush the fillets with melted butter, and sprinkle with the prepared spice mix until well coated.
4. Arrange the prepared fillets in a single layer, and place in the fryer's basket. Set the frying time to 10 minutes, and then let it cook until fork-tender, turning halfway and spraying with oil.
5. Serve immediately.

#40 Mullet with Garlic Oil (Air Fryer)

Preparation Time: 10 minutes/Cooking Time: 10 Minutes/Serves: 4 Servings (4 fillets per serving)

Nutrition Per Serving: Carbohydrates: 1.5 grams/Fat: 41.5 grams/Protein: 55.8 grams/Fiber: 0.05 grams/Calories: 605

Ingredients

- 4 whole mullets, gutted, cleaned
- 2 teaspoons salt
- 2 teaspoon ground black pepper
- Non-stick cooking oil spray
  For the Garlic Oil:
- 2 fillets of anchovy
- 3 cloves of garlic, peeled, chopped
- ½ tablespoon red chili flakes
- 1 tablespoon parsley leaves, chopped
- 2 tablespoons sunflower oil
- 1/3 cup olive oil

Directions

1. Switch on the air fryer and grease its frying basket with oil. Insert it into the fryer and close the cover. Select the cooking temperature up to 400 degrees F and preheat.
2. Prepare the fillet. Season with salt, and black pepper.

3. Arrange the prepared fillets in a single layer in the fryer's basket. Set the frying time to 10 minutes, and then let it cook until fork-tender, turning halfway and spraying with oil.
4. While still frying the fish, prepare the garlic oil. Use a small saucepan and place it over medium heat. Add chili flakes, anchovy, and sunflower oil.
5. Stir until well combined. Cook for 7 to 10 minutes until anchovy melts. Remove the pan from heat. Add olive oil, stir until mixed and let it cool until needed.
6. Stir parsley into the garlic oil. Scoop it evenly on four plates and add a fried fillet to each, and then serve.

#41 Mullet with Lemon and Caper Sauce (Air Fryer)

Preparation Time: 10 minutes/Cooking Time: 10 Minutes/Serves: 4 Servings (2 fillets per serving)

Nutrition Per Serving: Carbohydrates: 4.8 grams/Fat: 42 grams/Protein: 60.7 grams/Fiber: 1.3 grams/Calories: 640

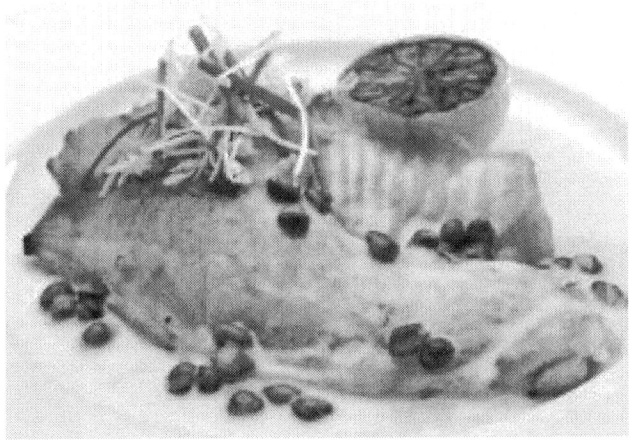

Ingredients

- 8 fillets of mullet, skin on, each about 4 ounces
- 4 teaspoons salt
- 4 teaspoons ground black pepper
- ¼ cup olive oil
  For the Lemon and Caper Sauce:
- 2 shallots, peeled, diced

- 2 lemons, juiced
- 2 tablespoons capers, rinsed
- 1/3 cup olive oil
- 2 tablespoons parsley leaves, chopped

Directions

1. Switch on the air fryer and grease its frying basket with oil. Insert it into the fryer and close the cover. Select the cooking temperature up to 400 degrees F and preheat.
2. Prepare the fillet. Brush the fillets with oil, and then season with salt, and black pepper.
3. Arrange the prepared fillets in a single layer. Place in the fryer's basket and set the frying time to 10 minutes. Let it cook until fork-tender, turning halfway and spraying with oil.
4. While still frying the fish, prepare the sauce using a medium bowl. Place all ingredients, and stir until well combined, and then set aside.
5. Divide the fillets into four plates, drizzle with the prepared lemon, and caper sauce. Serve with a green salad.

#42 Mullet with Tomato Sauce (Pan)

Preparation Time: 10 minutes/Cooking Time: 40 Minutes/Serves: 4 Servings (2 fillets with tomato sauce per serving)

Nutrition Per Serving: Carbohydrates: 18.2 grams/Fat: 38.2 grams/Protein: 62.8 grams/Fiber: 3.6 grams/Calories: 662

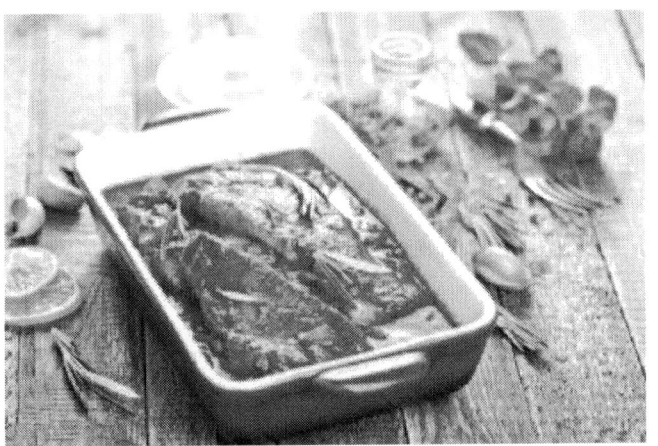

Ingredients

- 8 fillets of mullet, each about 4 ounces
- 2 tablespoons all-purpose flour
- 14 ounces canned tomatoes
- 2 medium white onion, peeled, sliced
- 2 small carrots, peeled, sliced
- 2 teaspoons minced garlic
- ½ of a lemon, juiced
- 1 ½ teaspoon salt

- 1 bay leaf
- 1 teaspoon ground black pepper
- 2 teaspoons tomato paste
- 1 cup dry white wine
- ½ cup olive oil, and more as needed to drizzle
- 2 tablespoons chopped parsley

Directions

1. Place fillets in a shallow dish, and, sprinkle with flour, salt, and black pepper. Toss until coated.
2. Using a large frying pan, place it over medium-high heat, and add ¼ cup oil.
3. Add fish fillets in a single layer, and then cook per side for 3 minutes until golden.
4. Transfer fried fillets to a plate, and then repeat with the remaining fillets. Set aside.
5. Clean and wipe the pan. Switch heat to a low level and add remaining oil. When pan is hot, add carrot, garlic, and onion. Cook the vegetables for 5 minutes, or until softened.
6. Add tomatoes and bay leaf and pour in tomato paste and wine. Stir until mixed, and then simmer for 15 minutes.
7. Return fried fillets into the pan, toss lightly until coated in the sauce. Continue cooking for 5 minutes.
8. When done, transfer fillets and tomato sauce to a serving dish, and let it cool for 10 minutes.
9. Drizzle with lemon juice, garnish with parsley leaves, and then serve.

NATHALIE SEATON

Oysters

#43 Oysters with Spicy Butter (Instant Pot)

Preparation Time: 10 minutes/Cooking Time: 2 Minutes/Serves: 20 Servings (1 oyster per serving)

Nutrition Per Serving: Carbohydrates: 4.6 grams/Fat: 7.2 grams/Protein: 3.5 grams/Fiber: 0.1 grams/Calories: 97.4

Ingredients

- 20 oysters in shells, fresh, scrubbed, rinsed
- ½ teaspoon dried parsley
- 2 teaspoons hot sauce
- 4 tablespoons butter, unsalted, melted
- 1 cup of water

Directions

1. Plug in the 4-quarts instant pot and pour water into the inner pot. Insert a trivet stand, or steamer basket, and then arrange the oyster on it.
2. Close the cover of the instant pot securely. Press the manual button and select the high-pressure setting. Set the cooking time to 2 minutes, and let it cook. The instant pot will take 5 to 10 minutes to build pressure, and then the cooking timer will start.

3. Place melted butter in a medium-sized bowl. Add parsley, and hot sauce. Stir until well combined.
4. When the instant pot beeps, quickly release the pressure. Open it, and then remove the oyster shells from it.
5. Use a spoon to open the oyster shells. Arrange them on a large plate, and top with the prepared butter mixture.
6. Serve right away.

#44 Oyster Stew (Instant Pot)

Preparation Time: 10 minutes/Cooking Time: 11 Minutes/Serves: 4 Servings (1 bowl per serving)

Nutrition Per Serving: Carbohydrates: 13 grams/Fat: 53 grams/Protein: 17 grams/Fiber: 1 grams/Calories: 597

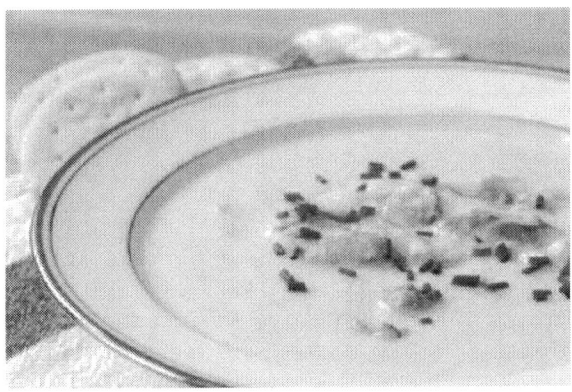

Ingredients

- 20 ounces oysters, without shell
- 2 tablespoons minced shallot
- 1 cup minced celery
- 1 teaspoon minced garlic
- ½ teaspoon of sea salt
- ¼ teaspoon ground white pepper
- 2 tablespoons butter, unsalted
- 1 ½ cup chicken broth
- 2 cups heavy cream or coconut milk, unsweetened
- 2 tablespoons fresh parsley, chopped

Directions

1. Plug in the 4-quarts instant pot and press the sauté button.
2. Add butter into the inner pot, and let it melt. Add celery, garlic, and shallot, and stir until mixed. Cook for 5 minutes.
3. Add oysters and pour in broth and cream. Stir until mixed, and then press the cancel button.
4. Close the cover of the instant pot securely. Press the manual button and select the low-pressure setting. Set the cooking time to 6 minutes. The instant pot will take 5 to 10 minutes to build pressure, and then the cooking timer will start.
5. When the instant pot beeps, quickly release the pressure, open it and stir in salt and black pepper.
6. Remove oysters from the instant pot, cut them with kitchen shears, and then put them back to the instant pot.
7. Distribute the oyster stew to 4 bowls, garnish with parsley, and then serve.

#45 Three-Cheese Baked Oysters (Oven)

Preparation Time: 10 minutes/Cooking Time: 10 Minutes/Serves: 14 Servings (1 oyster per serving)

Nutrition Per Serving: Carbohydrates: 0 grams/Fat: 7 grams/Protein: 3 grams/Fiber: 0 grams/Calories: 83

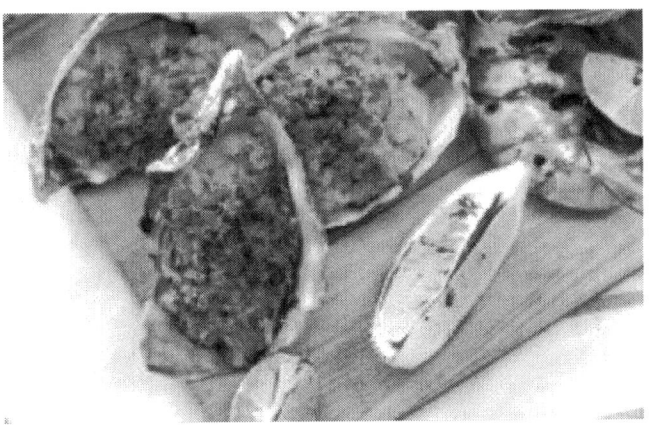

Ingredients

- 14 oysters in shells, fresh, scrubbed, rinsed
  The Stuffing:
- 1/3 cup cooked crumbled bacon
- ½ teaspoon minced garlic
- ¼ cup chopped spinach, frozen
- ¼ teaspoon red pepper flakes
- 2/3 cup shredded cheddar cheese
- 1/3 cup grated Parmesan cheese
- 5 ounces cream cheese, softened

Directions

1. Switch on the oven, then set it to 450 degrees F and preheat.
2. Open the oyster by using an oyster shucking knife. Remove the top shell, and then release the oyster from its shell by running the knife along with it, leaving the oyster in the bottom half of the shell.
3. Thaw the spinach and squeeze it to remove excess liquid. Place it in a medium bowl.
4. Add the remaining ingredients for the filling except for parmesan. Stir until combined, and then top it over oysters.
5. Arrange the oysters on a large baking sheet. Sprinkle parmesan cheese on top, and then bake for 8 to 10 minutes until cheese turn golden.
6. Serve right away.

NATHALIE SEATON

#46 Air Fried Oysters (Air Fryer)

Preparation Time: 10 minutes/Cooking Time: 8 Minutes/Serves: 4 Servings (4 oysters per serving)

Nutrition Per Serving: Carbohydrates: 11.6 grams/Fat: 4.6 grams/Protein: 18.9 grams/Fiber: 2 grams/Calories: 169.1

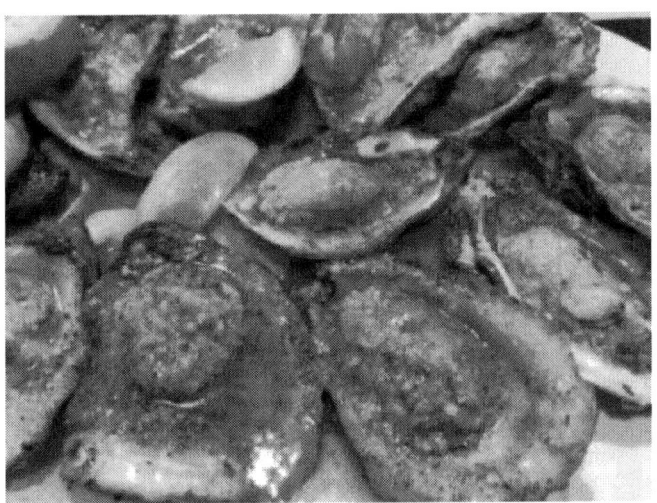

Ingredients

- 16 oysters in half-shells, fresh, scrubbed, rinsed
- 1 tablespoon hot pepper sauce
- 2 tablespoons Worcestershire sauce

Directions

1. Switch on the air fryer and grease its frying basket with oil. Insert it into the fryer and close the cover. Select the cooking temperature up to 400 degrees F and preheat.
2. Arrange the oysters in a half shell by single layer. Place in the fryer's basket and set the frying time to 4 minutes. Let it cook.
3. When done, transfer oysters to a serving plate, and then drizzle with hot pepper sauce, and Worcestershire sauce.
4. Repeat with the remaining oysters, and then serve.

NATHALIE SEATON

#47 Breaded Oysters (Air Fryer)

Preparation Time: 25 minutes/Cooking Time: 12 Minutes/Serves: 3 Servings (4 oysters per serving)

Nutrition Per Serving: Carbohydrates: 29.4 grams/Fat: 5.6 grams/Protein: 9.1 grams/Fiber: 2 grams/Calories: 203

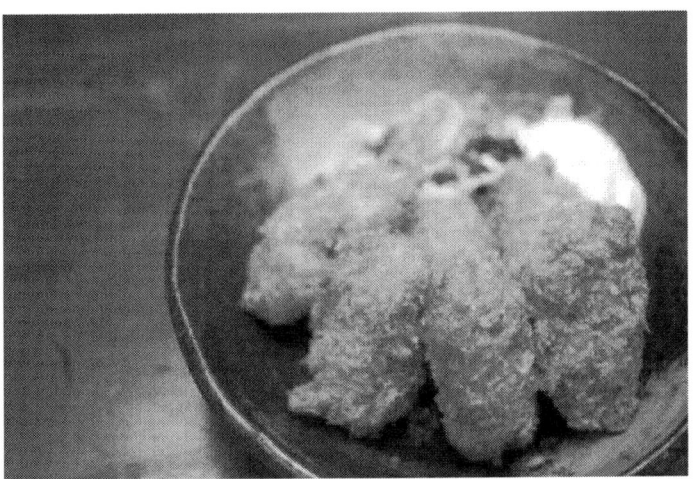

Ingredients

- 12 fresh oysters, without shell
- 1 cup panko breadcrumbs
- ½ teaspoon salt
- ½ cup all-purpose flour
- ½ tsp Cajun seasoning
- ½ teaspoon ground black pepper
- 3 tablespoons hot sauce
- 2 eggs
- Non-stick cooking oil spray

Directions

1. Crack the eggs in a shallow dish. Add hot sauce and whisk until blended.
2. Place flour, and breadcrumbs in two separate shallow dishes.
3. Use a large baking sheet, and line it with a parchment sheet.
4. Work on one oyster at a time, and pat dry with paper towels. Lightly coat in flour, and dip into the egg mixture. Toss in breadcrumbs until coated.
5. Arrange the prepared oyster on the baking sheet and repeat with the remaining oysters. Refrigerate for a minimum of 15 minutes.
6. When ready to cook, switch on the air fryer, and grease its frying basket with oil. Insert it into the fryer and close the cover. Select the cooking temperature up to 400 degrees F and preheat.
7. Arrange the oysters in a single layer and place in the fryer's basket. Spray with oil and set the frying time to 6 minutes. Let it cook, flipping oysters halfway and spraying with oil.
8. When done, transfer oysters to a serving plate, and then repeat with the remaining oysters.
9. Serve right away.

#48 Almond and Cheese Crusted Oysters (Air Fryer)

Preparation Time: 10 minutes/Cooking Time: 12 Minutes/Serves: 3 Servings (4 oysters per serving)

Nutrition Per Serving: Carbohydrates: 1 grams/Fat: 2 grams/Protein: 1 grams/Fiber: 0.1 grams/Calories: 112

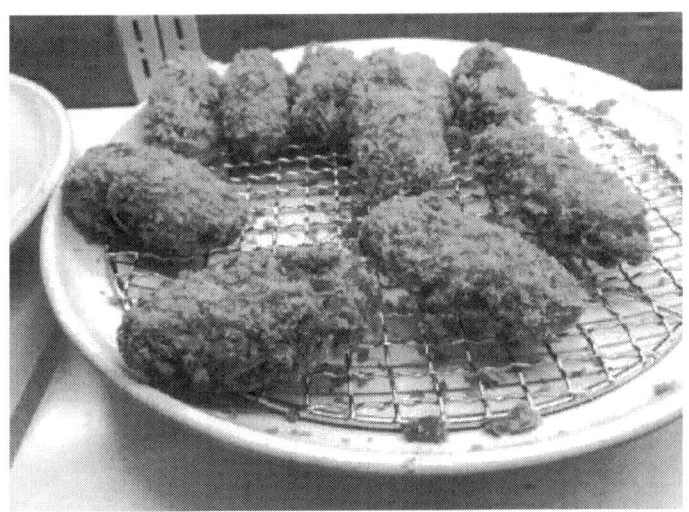

Ingredients

- 12 fresh oysters, without shell
- ¼ cup almond flour
- ½ teaspoon salt
- 1 egg
- ¼ cup grated Parmesan cheese
- Non-stick cooking oil spray

Directions

1. Place the flour in a shallow dish. Add cheese, and then stir until mixed.
2. In another shallow dish, crack the egg, and then whisk until blended.
3. When ready to cook, switch on the air fryer, and grease its frying basket with oil. Insert it into the fryer. Close the cover and select the cooking temperature up to 400 degrees F and preheat.
4. Work on one oyster at a time, and pat dry with a paper towel. Lightly coat in almond flour mixture. Dip into the egg, and then cover again in almond flour mixture until thoroughly coated.
5. Arrange the prepared oysters in a single layer. Place in the fryer basket, and spray with oil. Set the frying time to 6 minutes, and then let it cook, flipping oysters halfway and spraying with oil.
6. When done, transfer oysters to a serving plate, and then repeat with the remaining oysters.
7. Serve right away.

NATHALIE SEATON

Pollock

#49 Coconut Crusted Pollock (Instant Pot)

Preparation Time: 10 minutes/Cooking Time: 3 Minutes/Serves: 3 Servings (1 fish fillet and 1/3-pound asparagus per serving)

Nutrition Per Serving: Carbohydrates: 83 grams/Fat: 23 grams/Protein: 38 grams/Fiber: 11 grams/Calories: 672

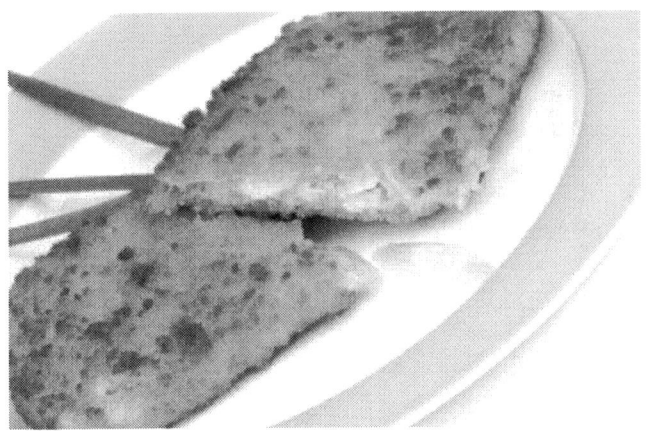

Ingredients

- 3 fillets of Pollock, each about 4 to 6 ounces
- 1-pound asparagus
- ½ teaspoon salt
- ½ teaspoon ground black pepper

- 3 lemons, cut into slices
- 2 tablespoons butter, unsalted
- ½ cup of water

For the Coconut Crust:
- ½ cup coconut flakes, unsweetened
- ½ teaspoon salt
- ½ teaspoon garlic powder
- ¼ teaspoon ground pepper
- 1 teaspoon cumin
- ½ cup panko breadcrumbs
- 2 tablespoons honey
- 2 eggs

Directions

1. Switch on the 4-quarts instant pot and pour water into the inner pot. Insert a trivet stand, or a steamer basket, and then layer it with asparagus.
2. Close the cover of the instant pot securely. Press the manual button and select the high-pressure setting. Set the cooking time to 10 minutes, and let it cook. The instant pot will take 5 to 10 minutes to build pressure, and then the cooking timer will start.
3. When the instant pot beeps, quickly release the pressure, open it and then transfer asparagus to a plate.
4. Top asparagus with butter, sprinkle with salt and black pepper. Toss until coated, and then set aside until needed.

5. Prepare the fish. Crack the eggs in a shallow dish. Add honey, and then whisk until combined.
6. Use another shallow dish, and place the remaining ingredients for the breading, and then stir until combined.
7. Work on one fillet at a time. Dip into the egg mixture, and then lightly coat in coconut mixture until thoroughly covered.
8. Arrange the fillets on the steamer rack. Top with 1 to 2 slices of lemon, and then close the cover of the instant pot.
9. Press the manual button and select the high-pressure setting. Set the cooking time to 3 minutes, and let it cook. The instant pot will take 5 to 10 minutes to build pressure, and then the cooking timer will start.
10. When the instant pot beeps, quickly release the pressure, open it, and then transfer fillet to serving plates.
11. Serve the coconut-crusted fillets with asparagus.

#50 Pollock with Cheesy-Herb Crust (Air Fryer)

Preparation Time: 10 minutes/Cooking Time: 12 Minutes/Serves: 4 Servings (1 fillet per serving)

Nutrition Per Serving: Carbohydrates: 7 grams/Fat: 22.4 grams/Protein: 43.4 grams/Fiber: 0.4 grams/Calories: 406

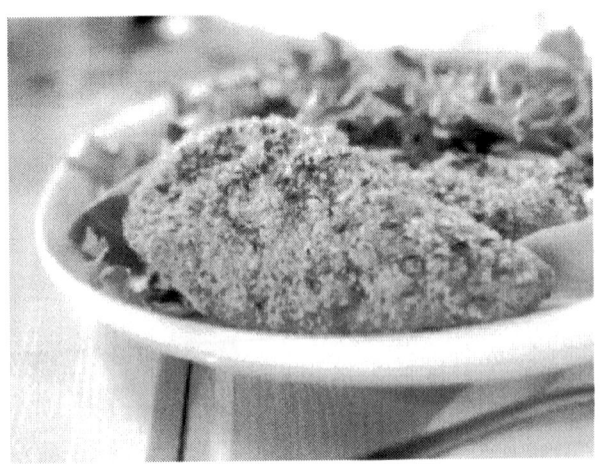

Ingredients

- 4 fillets of Pollock, each about 4 to 6 ounces, skin-on
- 1 teaspoon salt
- ½ teaspoon ground black pepper
- Non-stick cooking oil spray
  For the Breading:
- 1/3 cup breadcrumbs

- ½ teaspoon salt
- ¼ teaspoon ground black pepper
- ¼ cup grated cheddar cheese
- 4 tablespoons chopped parsley
- 1 tablespoon chopped dill
- ½ teaspoon minced garlic
- 4 tablespoons butter, unsalted, melted

Directions

1. Prepare the fillets. Coat with oil, and then season with salt and black pepper. Switch on the air fryer and grease its frying basket with oil. Insert it into the fryer and close the cover. Select the cooking temperature up to 400 degrees F and preheat.
2. Using a shallow dish, place all the ingredients for the breading, and then stir until well combined.
3. Work on one fillet at a time, lightly coat and press the fillet into the breadcrumbs' mixture.
4. Arrange the prepared fillets in a single layer in the fryer basket. Set the frying time to 12 minutes, and then let it cook, turning halfway.
5. Serve right away.

#51 Crispy Pollock with Tartar Sauce (Air Fryer)

Preparation Time: 10 minutes/Cooking Time: 12 Minutes/Serves: 4 Servings

Nutrition Per Serving: Carbohydrates: 26.4 grams/Fat: 22 grams/Protein: 35.2 grams/Fiber: 1.6 grams/Calories: 440

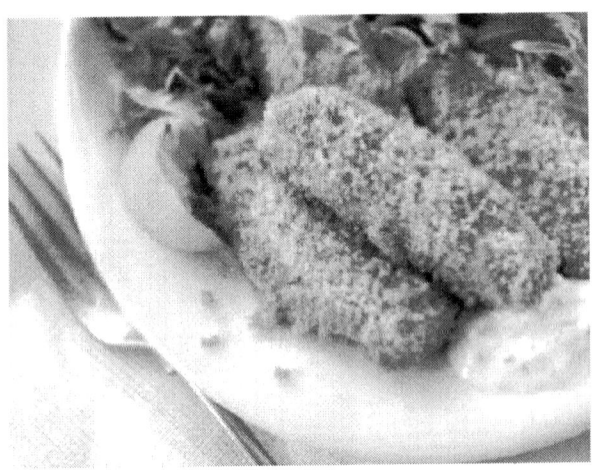

Ingredients

- 1 ¼ pound Pollock fillets
- 1 teaspoon salt
- 1 teaspoon ground black pepper
- Non-stick cooking oil spray
  For the Breading:
- 1/3 cup all-purpose flour

- ½ teaspoon salt
- ½ teaspoon ground black pepper
- 1 ½ cup potato flakes
- 2 eggs

For the Tartar Sauce:
- 1 tablespoon capers
- 2 tablespoons sweet pickle relish
- 1 tablespoon vinegar
- ¼ cup mayonnaise

Directions

1. Cut the fillets into long sticks. Season them with salt and black pepper.
2. Switch on the air fryer and grease its frying basket with oil. Insert it into the fryer and close the cover. Select the cooking temperature up to 400 degrees F and preheat.
3. Crack the eggs in a shallow dish and add salt and black pepper. Whisk until beaten.
4. Use a separate dish and place flour in it. Get another shallow dish and place the potato flake.
5. Work on one fillet at a time, and lightly coat into the flour. Dip into the egg and then coat with the potato flakes.
6. Arrange the prepared fillets in a single layer in the fryer basket. Set the frying time to 12 minutes, and then let it cook, turning halfway and coating with oil.

7. While fillets are frying, prepare the tartar sauce. Use a small bowl, and place all ingredients, and then stir until well combined.
8. When done frying, transfer to a serving dish, season with salt and black pepper, and then serve together with the tartar sauce.

#52 Sautéed Pollock with Parmesan Crumbs (Pan)

Preparation Time: 10 minutes/Cooking Time: 12 Minutes/Serves: 4 Servings (1 fillet per serving)

Nutrition Per Serving: Carbohydrates: 16 grams/Fat: 13 grams/Protein: 24 grams/Fiber: 2 grams/Calories: 270

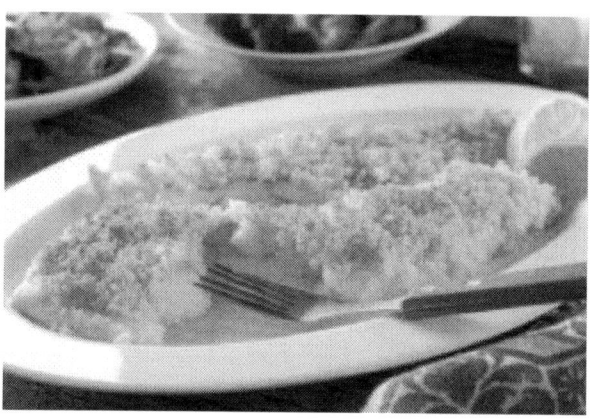

Ingredients

- 4 fillets of Pollock, each about 4 to 6 ounces
- 2/3 cup panko breadcrumbs
- 1 teaspoon salt
- 1 teaspoon ground black pepper
- 3 tablespoons chopped parsley
- ¼ teaspoon cayenne pepper
- 1/3 cup grated parmesan cheese
- 3 tablespoons olive oil
- 1 lemon, cut into wedges

Directions

1. Place a large skillet pan over medium-high heat and add breadcrumbs. Cook for 2 to 3 minutes until light brown.
2. Transfer the breadcrumbs to a shallow dish. Add salt, black pepper, parsley, cayenne pepper, 1 tablespoon oil, and cheese, and then stir until well combined.
3. Wipe clean the pan, and place over medium-high heat. Add remaining oil, and when hot, add fillets.
4. Cook the fillets for 5 minutes, flip the other side, and then top with a generous amount of breadcrumbs mixture.
5. Cover the pan with its lid, and then cook for 5 minutes.
6. Serve right away.

#53 Lemon-Dill Pollock (Air Fryer)

Preparation Time: 20 minutes/Cooking Time: 12 Minutes/Serves: 4 Servings (1 fillet per serving)

Nutrition Per Serving: Carbohydrates: 1.4 grams/Fat: 3.7 grams/Protein: 33.2 grams/Fiber: 0.1 grams/Calories: 180

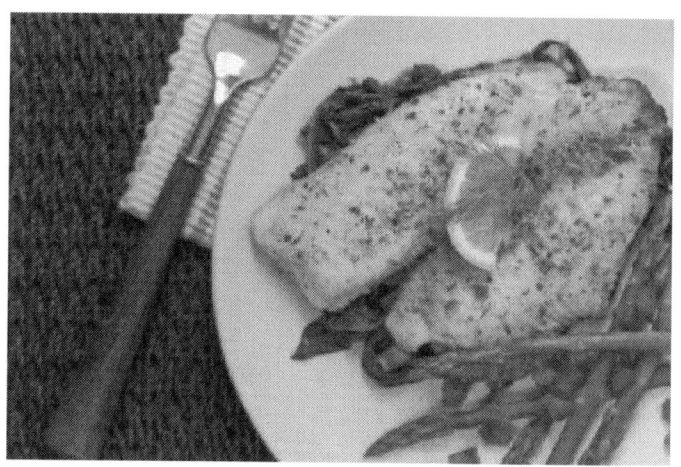

Ingredients

- 4 fillets of Pollock, each about 4 to 6 ounces
- Non-stick cooking oil spray
  For the Marinade:
- 4 teaspoons Dijon mustard
- ⅓ cup minced dill
- ½ teaspoon minced garlic
- ¼ teaspoon salt

- ¼ cup lemon juice
- ¼ teaspoon ground black pepper
- ¼ teaspoon sugar
- 1 tablespoon olive oil

Directions

1. Place all the ingredients for the marinade in a medium bowl. Stir until combined, and then pour into a large plastic bag.
2. Add fillets into the bag, seal it, and turn it upside down to coat fillets with the marinade. Marinate for 15 minutes. Refrigerate.
3. When ready to cook, switch on the air fryer, and grease its frying basket with oil. Insert it into the fryer and close the cover. Select the cooking temperature up to 400 degrees and preheat.
4. Arrange the prepared fillets in a single layer in the fryer basket, and spray with oil. Set the frying time to 12 minutes, and let it cook until fork tender, turning halfway and coating with oil.
5. Serve right away.

#54 Mediterranean Spice Pollock (Air Fryer)

Preparation Time: 10 minutes/Cooking Time: 12 Minutes/Serves: 4 Servings (1/4-pound fillet per serving)

Nutrition Per Serving: Carbohydrates: 1.1 grams/Fat: 13.4 grams/Protein: 80.7 grams/Fiber: 0.3 grams/Calories: 449

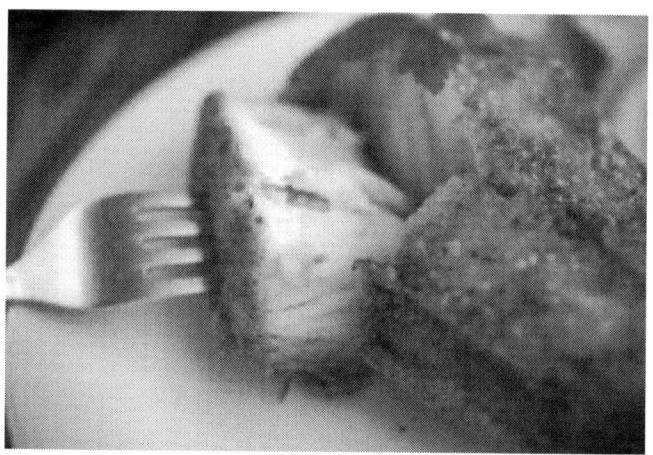

Ingredients

- 1-pound Pollock fillets
- 1 lemon, cut into wedges
- 2 tablespoons parsley leaves, chopped
  For the Seasoning:
- 1 teaspoon minced garlic
- ¼ teaspoon salt

- 1 teaspoon dried rosemary
- ½ teaspoon dried oregano
- ¼ teaspoon ground black pepper
- 1 teaspoon ground cumin
- ½ teaspoon paprika
- 1 teaspoon ground coriander
- ¼ teaspoon ground cinnamon
- 3 tablespoons olive oil

Directions

1. Switch on the air fryer and grease its frying basket with oil. Insert it into the fryer and close the cover. Select the cooking temperature up to 375 degrees F and preheat.
2. Using a small bowl, place all the ingredients for the seasoning. Stir until combined, and then spread the mixture on fillets until evenly coated.
3. Arrange the prepared fillets in a single layer and place in the fryer's basket. Set the frying time to 12 minutes, and then let it cook until fork-tender, turning halfway.
4. When done, garnish the fillet with parsley, and then serve with lemon wedges.

NATHALIE SEATON

Sardines

#55 Lentil and Vegetable Soup with Sardine (Instant Pot)

Preparation Time: 10 minutes/Cooking Time: 20 Minutes/Serves: 4 Servings (1 bowl per serving)

Nutrition Per Serving: Carbohydrates: 41 grams/Fat: 9.6 grams/Protein: 17.6 grams/Fiber: 8 grams/Calories: 322

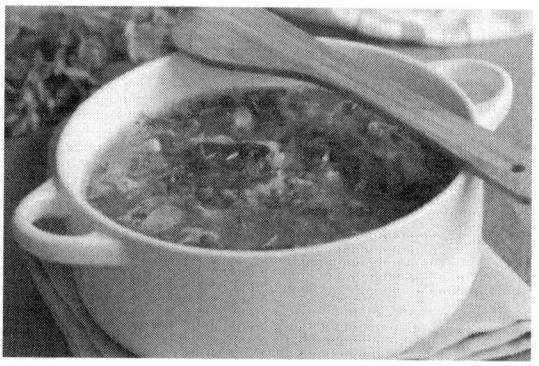

Ingredients

- 3.75 ounces canned sardines, skinless, boneless, packed in oil
- 1 cup brown lentils
- 1¾ cups diced zucchini
- 1 cup diced onion
- 1 cup sliced carrots
- 3 small tomatoes, quartered
- 1 celery stalk, trimmed, ¼-inch dice

- 1 teaspoon minced garlic
- ½ teaspoon salt
- ¼ teaspoon ground black pepper
- ⅛ teaspoon red chili powder
- 1 teaspoon ground cumin
- ½ teaspoon ground turmeric
- 2 tablespoons olive oil
- 4 cups vegetable broth

Directions

1. Switch on the 4-quarts instant pot and press the sauté button. Add oil when it is hot.
2. Add zucchini, celery, carrot, and onion. Then cook for 5 minutes until vegetables turn soft.
3. Stir in garlic, salt, black pepper, red chili powder, turmeric, and cumin. Continue cooking for 2 minutes.
4. Add tomatoes and lentils, pour in the broth, and stir until well combined. Press the cancel button.
5. Close the cover of the instant pot securely. Press the manual button and select the high-pressure setting. Set the cooking time to 10 minutes, and let it cook. The instant pot will take 5 to 8 minutes to build pressure, and then the cooking timer will start.
6. When the instant pot beeps, quickly release the pressure, and open the instant pot carefully.
7. Drain the sardines, and then break into bite-size pieces. Add to the soup and stir until mixed. Let the soup rest for 5 minutes.
8. Place the soup in serving bowls, and then serve.

#56 Sweet and Sour Fish (Instant Pot)

Preparation Time: 10 minutes/Cooking Time: 15 Minutes/Serves: 3 Servings

Nutrition Per Serving: Carbohydrates: 28.7 grams/Fat: 32.6 grams/Protein: 57.4 grams/Fiber: 1.1 grams/Calories: 638

Ingredients

- 8 whole sardines, fresh, gutted, cleaned
- 2 shallots, peeled, sliced
- 2 tablespoons chopped ginger
- 2 teaspoons minced garlic
- 2 green chilies, chopped
- 1 tablespoon salt
- 1/3 cup sugar
- ½ teaspoon ground black pepper
- 2 bay leaves
- 2 tablespoons olive oil
- ¼ cup vinegar
- 1 ½ cup water
- 1 green onion, sliced

Directions

1. Prepare the sardines. Remove its insides, rinse well until thoroughly clean, and then pat dry with paper towels.
2. Switch on the 4-quarts instant pot and press the sauté button. add oil.
3. Add shallots, chilies, garlic, and ginger, stir until mixed, and then cook for 5 minutes until vegetables turn soft.
4. Press the cancel button, and then top with sardines in a single layer.
5. Add salt, black pepper, sugar, vinegar, and water in a small bowl, and whisk until combined. Pour the mixture over the fish and add bay leaves.
6. Close the cover of the instant pot securely. Press the manual button and select the high-pressure setting. Set the cooking time to 8 minutes, and let it cook. The instant pot will take 5 to 10 minutes to build pressure, and then the cooking timer will start.
7. When the instant pot beeps, quickly release the pressure, then carefully open the instant pot. Remove the bay leaves, and then garnish it with green onion.
8. Serve immediately.

#57 Mediterranean Sardine Pasta (Pan)

Preparation Time: 10 minutes/Cooking Time: 15 Minutes/Serves: 4 Servings

Nutrition Per Serving: Carbohydrates: 44 grams/Fat: 22 grams/Protein: 7 grams/Fiber: 2 grams/Calories: 404

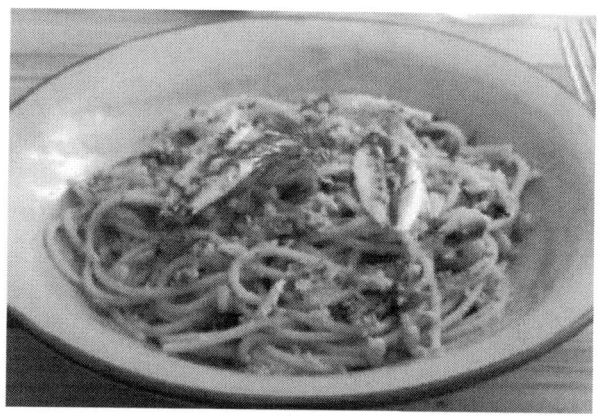

Ingredients

- 4.375 ounces canned sardines, skinless, boneless, packed in oil, drained
- ¼ cup minced shallots
- ½ teaspoon salt
- ½ teaspoon crushed red pepper flakes
- 2 teaspoons lemon zest
- 3 tablespoons capers, rinsed
- 5 tablespoons lemon juice
- 6 tablespoons olive oil
- 3 tablespoons fresh parsley, chopped
- 8 ounces of spaghetti, uncooked

PESCATARIAN COOKBOOK FOR BEGINNERS

Directions

1. Fill a large pot with half full water. Place it over high heat and bring it to a boil.
2. Add spaghetti and cook for 8 to 10 minutes until the pasta is tender. Drain it well, and reserve ½ cup of the pasta water.
3. While pasta cooks, get a large skillet pan and place it over medium heat, then add oil.
4. Add shallots, and stir in salt, red pepper flakes, and lemon zest. Cook for 3 to 4 minutes until shallots turn soft.
5. Add capers and sardines. Break sardines into pieces, and then cook for 2 minutes until sardines begin to turn golden.
6. Stir in lemon juice, and switch heat to low level and let it cook until the pasta is cooked.
7. Add cooked pasta into the skillet pan. Add parsley, and then toss until pasta is well mixed with the sauce.
8. If the pasta looks dry, add reserved pasta water, 1 tablespoon at a time. Then taste it to adjust seasoning.
9. Serve right away.

#58 Herb-Stuffed Sardines (Air Fryer)

Preparation Time: 10 minutes/Cooking Time: 30 Minutes/Serves: 3 Servings (2 sardines per serving)

Nutrition Per Serving: Carbohydrates: 5 grams/Fat: 36 grams/Protein: 20 grams/Fiber: 2 grams/Calories: 415

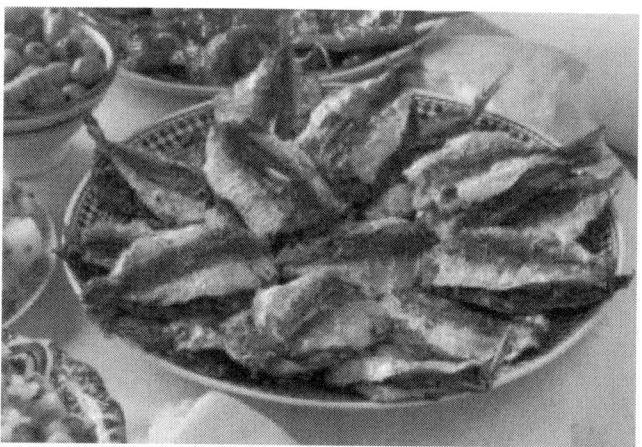

Ingredients

- 6 large sardines, about 2 pounds total, fresh, gutted, cleaned
- 4 green onions, chopped
- 1 teaspoon salt
- ½ teaspoon ground black pepper
- ½ cup parsley leaves, fresh
- 3 tablespoons butter, unsalted
- 2 tablespoons olive oil
- 1 lemon, cut into wedges

Directions

1. Prepare the sardines. Remove its insides, rinse them well until thoroughly clean, and then pat dry with paper towels.
2. Place butter in a food processor. Add green onions, parsley leaves, salt, and black pepper, and then press the pulse button until the mixture comes together.
3. Stuff each sardine with the butter-parsley mixture, and then brush the skin of sardines with oil.
4. Switch on the air fryer. Line the frying basket with foil, grease it with oil and insert it into the fryer. Close the cover and select the cooking temperature up to 390 degrees F and preheat.
5. Arrange the prepared sardines into the fryer's basket, and then fry for 15 minutes per side until golden brown, turning halfway.
6. Serve the sardines with lemon wedges.

NATHALIE SEATON

#59 Spicy Sardines (Air Fryer)

Preparation Time: 10 minutes/Cooking Time: 30 Minutes/Serves: 2 Servings (per serving)

Nutrition Per Serving: Carbohydrates: 1.9 grams/Fat: 47.8 grams/Protein: 86 grams/Fiber: 0.5 grams/Calories: 783

Ingredients

- 8 whole sardines, fresh, gutted, cleaned
- Non-stick cooking oil spray
  For the Marinade:
- 2 tablespoons red chili powder
- 1 teaspoon turmeric powder
- 1 teaspoon salt
- 1 tablespoon garlic powder
- 3 tablespoons water

Directions

1. Prepare the sardines. Remove its head, tail, and insides, and make few cuts on each side of the fish. Rinse it well until thoroughly clean, and then pat dry with paper towels.
2. Prepare the marinade. Use a small bowl and place all ingredients, and then stir until combined.
3. Rub the marinade to the whole sardines until well coated, and then set aside until needed.
7. Meanwhile, switch on the air fryer, and grease the fryer's basket with oil. Insert it into the fryer and

close the cover. Select the cooking temperature up to 390 degrees F and preheat.
8. Arrange the marinated sardines into the fryer's basket. Spray with oil and then fry for 15 minutes per side until thoroughly cooked, turning halfway and spraying with oil.
4. Serve right away.

#60 Fried Sardines with Parsley Caper Sauce (Air Fryer)

Preparation Time: 10 minutes/Cooking Time: 20 Minutes/Serves: 4 Servings (3 sardines per serving)

Nutrition Per Serving: Carbohydrates: 19.7 grams/Fat: 39 grams/Protein: 71.6 grams/Fiber: 0.7 grams/Calories: 718

Ingredients

- 12 whole sardines, fresh, gutted, cleaned
- 1 teaspoon salt
- ½ cup all-purpose flour
- ½ teaspoon ground black pepper
- 1 cup panko breadcrumbs
- 2 eggs
- Non-stick cooking oil spray
  For the Sauce:
- 1 teaspoon capers
- ½ teaspoon salt
- ½ teaspoon ground black pepper
- 2 tablespoons lemon juice
- ½ cup olive oil
- 1 egg yolk
- 1/3 cup chopped parsley leaves

Directions

1. Sauce preparation: Place capers, lemon juice, and yolks in a medium bowl, and then press the pulse button of hand blender until smooth.
2. Slowly blend in oil, salt, black pepper, and parsley until almost combined, then cover the bowl with its lid, and refrigerate until needed.
3. Prepare the sardines. Remove its head, tail, and insides, rinse it well until thoroughly clean, and then pat dry with paper towels.
4. Place flour in a medium bowl, add salt and black pepper, and then stir until mixed.
5. Scoop the flour mixture into a large plastic bag, add 3 to 4 sardines. Seal the bag and then shake well until fully coated.
6. Switch on the air fryer and grease the fryer's basket with oil. Insert it into the fryer and close the cover. Select the cooking temperature up to 450 degrees F and preheat.
7. Crack the eggs in a shallow dish, and then whisk until blended.
8. Get another shallow dish, and then spread breadcrumbs in it.
9. Work on one sardine at a time. Dip in egg, and then lightly cover in breadcrumbs until coated.
10. Arrange the prepared sardines into the fryer's basket. Spray with oil, and then fry for 10 minutes per side until thoroughly cooked, turning halfway and spraying with oil.
11. Serve the sardines with the prepared sauce.

Salmon

#61 Salmon Scrambled Eggs (Pan)

Preparation Time: 10 minutes/Cooking Time: 6 Minutes/Serves: 2 Servings (1 toast with scrambled egg per serving)

Nutrition Per Serving: Carbohydrates: 24.5 grams/Fat: 27.24 grams/Protein: 27.2 grams/Fiber: 3.3 grams/Calories: 454

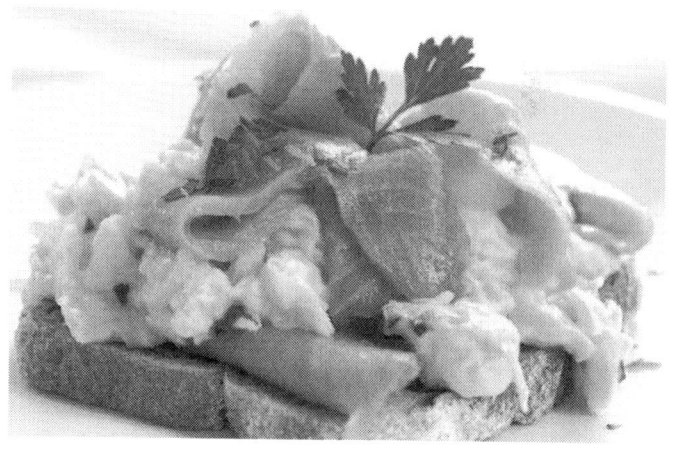

Ingredients

- 2 ounces sliced smoked salmon
- 1/8 teaspoon salt
- 1/8 teaspoon ground black pepper

- 2 teaspoons chopped chives
- 1 tablespoon butter, unsalted
- 3 tablespoons heavy cream
- 4 eggs
- 2 slices of whole-wheat bread

Directions

1. Set aside a slice of smoked salmon, and then chop the remaining smoked salmon.
2. Crack the eggs in a large bowl. Add 1 teaspoon chives, salt, and black pepper, and then whisk until blended.
3. Place a large skillet pan over medium heat, then add butter, and let it melt.
4. When the butter has melted, pour in the egg batter, and cook with a wooden spoon until eggs have scrambled to the desired level. The eggs should remain wet, not dry.
5. Then add chopped smoked salmon and stir until mixed. Remove the pan from heat and place it on a trivet stand.
6. Top the eggs with the remaining smoked salmon, and then garnish with the remaining chives.
7. When serving, toast the bread slices until golden brown, and slightly crisp. Then top the salmon scrambled egg generously.

#62 Teriyaki Salmon (Oven)

Preparation Time: 10 minutes/Cooking Time: 20 Minutes/Serves: 4 Servings (1 salmon fillet per serving)

Nutrition Per Serving: Carbohydrates: 24 grams/Fat: 10 grams/Protein: 35 grams/Fiber: 7 grams/Calories: 340

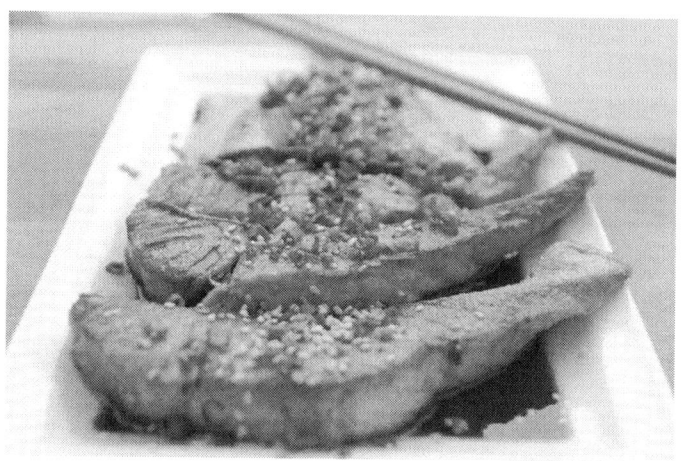

Ingredients

- 4 salmon fillets, skinless, each fillet about 6 ounces
- 1 tablespoon corn starch
- 1 tablespoon olive oil
- 2 tablespoons water
- 1 green onion, green part chopped
- ½ teaspoon sesame seeds
  For the Sauce:

- 1 tablespoon minced garlic
- 1 tablespoon grated ginger
- 2 tablespoons brown sugar
- 6 tablespoons soy sauce, low sodium
- 3 tablespoons honey
- 1 ½ tablespoon lemon juice
- 6 tablespoons water

Directions

1. Switch on the oven, then set it up to 400 degrees F and preheat.
2. Use a large baking dish that is large enough to fill fillets. Brush with oil, and then set aside.
3. To make a sauce, get a small saucepan, and place all ingredients, and then whisk until mixed.
4. Place the saucepan over medium heat, and then bring the sauce to a light boil.
5. Meanwhile, place cornstarch and water in a small bowl. Stir until smooth.
6. When the sauce comes to a boil, whisk the cornstarch mixture into the sauce. Let it boil for 1 minute, whisking continuously.
7. Remove the saucepan from heat and let it cool for 5 minutes.
8. Arrange the salmon slices in the prepared baking dish. Place the cooked sauce over fillets and then flip the other side so that fillets are coated in sauce completely.
9. Place the baking dish containing fillets into the oven, and then bake for 12 to 15 minutes until salmon has thoroughly cooked.

10. When done, transfer salmon fillets to a serving dish, and drizzle some sauce from the baking dish over the fillets. Sprinkle chopped green onion and sesame seeds on top.
11. Serve right away.

#63 Fried Salmon with Mustard (Air Fryer)

Preparation Time: 10 minutes/Cooking Time: 10 Minutes/Serves: 2 Servings (1 fillet per serving)

Nutrition Per Serving: Carbohydrates: 7.1 grams/Fat: 25.8 grams/Protein: 37.7 grams/Fiber: 0.05 grams/Calories: 409

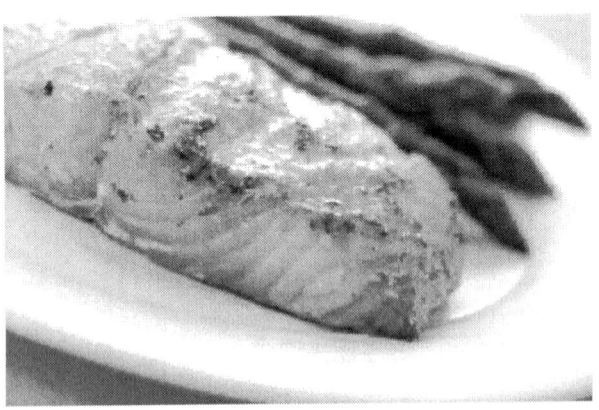

Ingredients

- 2 fillets of salmon, each about 6 ounces
- 1 teaspoon salt
- ½ teaspoon minced garlic
- 2 tablespoons Dijon mustard
- 1 tablespoon brown sugar
- ½ teaspoon dried thyme
- ½ teaspoon ground black pepper
- 2 teaspoons olive oil

Directions

1. Switch on the air fryer and grease the fryer's basket with oil. Insert it into the fryer and close the cover. Select the cooking temperature up to 400 degrees F and preheat.
2. Meanwhile, prepare the salmon by seasoning it with salt and black pepper.
3. Add garlic, sugar, mustard, thyme, and oil in a small bowl. Stir until combined, and then spread the mixture on top of salmon fillets.
4. Arrange the prepared salmon fillets into the fryer's basket, and then fry for 10 minutes until tender.
5. Serve right away.

#64 Salmon Cakes (Air Fryer)

Preparation Time: 10 minutes/Cooking Time: 12 Minutes/Serves: 2 Servings (2 salmon cakes per serving)

Nutrition Per Serving: Carbohydrates: 14.7 grams/Fat: 26.7 grams/Protein: 51.8 grams/Fiber: 2.1 grams/Calories: 517

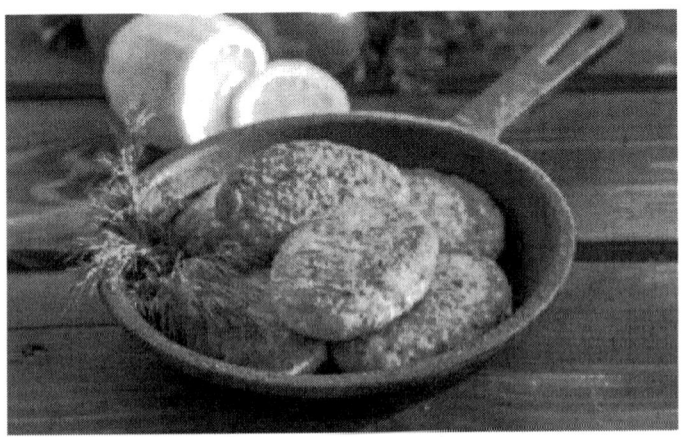

Ingredients

- 2 cans of pink salmon with bones and skin, unsalted, each about 7.5 ounce
- 2 tablespoons chopped fresh dill
- ¼ teaspoon ground black pepper
- ½ cup panko breadcrumbs
- 2 teaspoons Dijon mustard
- 2 tablespoons mayonnaise

- 1 egg
- 2 wedges of lemon
- Non-stick cooking oil spray

Directions

1. Switch on the air fryer and grease the fryer's basket with oil. Insert it into the fryer and close the cover. Select the cooking temperature up to 400 degrees F and preheat.
2. Meanwhile, drain the salmon. Remove the skin and bones, and then place in a medium bowl.
3. Add black pepper, dill, mustard, mayonnaise, breadcrumbs, and egg. Stir until well combined, and then shape the mixture into four patties.
4. Arrange the prepared salmon cakes into the fryer's basket. Spray with oil, and then fry for 12 minutes until golden brown on both sides, turning halfway and spraying with oil.
5. Serve the salmon cakes with lemon wedges.

PESCATARIAN COOKBOOK FOR BEGINNERS

#65 Honey Glazed Salmon (Air Fryer)

Preparation Time: 10 minutes/Cooking Time: 6 Minutes/Serves: 8 Servings (1 fillet per serving)

Nutrition Per Serving: Carbohydrates: 5 grams/Fat: 11 grams/Protein: 34 grams/Fiber: 2 grams/Calories: 262

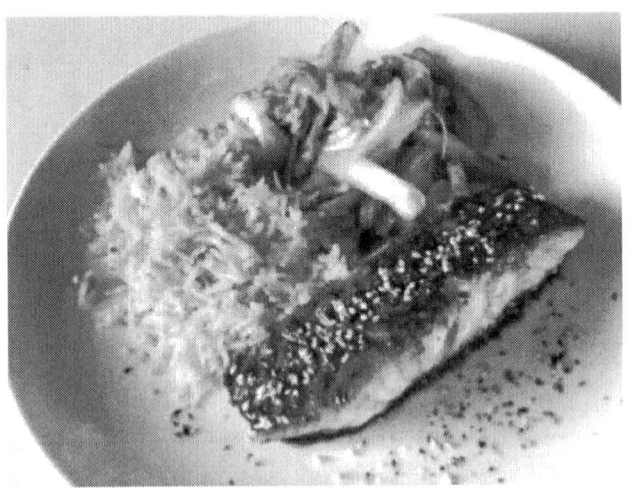

Ingredients

- 4 fillets of salmon, skin on, each about 4 to 6 ounces
- 1 teaspoon salt
- 1 teaspoon ground black pepper
- 1 tablespoon honey
- 2 teaspoons soy sauce
- 1 teaspoon sesame seeds

Directions

1. Switch on the air fryer and grease the fryer's basket with oil. Insert it into the fryer and close the cover. Select the cooking temperature up to 375 degrees F and preheat.
2. Meanwhile, season the salmon fillets with salt, and black pepper. Brush with soy sauce until coated.
3. Arrange the prepared salmon fillets into the fryer's basket, and then fry for 6 minutes until fork-tender, turning halfway.
4. Then brush each side of fillet with honey. Sprinkle with sesame seeds and continue frying for 2 minutes until done.
5. Serve right away.

PESCATARIAN COOKBOOK FOR BEGINNERS

#66 Sweet Spicy Salmon (Air Fryer)

Preparation Time: 10 minutes/Cooking Time: 12 Minutes/Serves: 3 Servings (1 fillet per serving)

Nutrition Per Serving: Carbohydrates: 23 grams/Fat: 11 grams/Protein: 34 grams/Fiber: 2 grams/Calories: 325

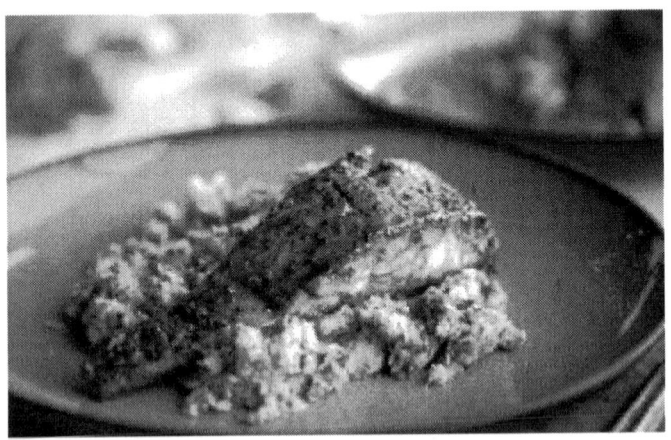

Ingredients

- 3 fillets of salmon, each about 4 to 6 ounces
- 1/8 teaspoon salt
- ½ teaspoon red chili powder
- 1/8 teaspoon ground black pepper
- 1 tablespoon red chili flakes
- ½ teaspoon turmeric powder
- ¼ cup honey
- 1 ½ teaspoon ground coriander

Directions

1. Switch on the air fryer and grease the fryer's basket with oil. Insert it into the fryer and close the cover. Select the cooking temperature up to 400 degrees F and preheat.
2. Meanwhile, get a small heatproof bowl, place honey in it. Microwave for 10 seconds until slightly warm.
3. Add salt, red chili powder, black pepper, red chili flakes, coriander, and turmeric powder. Stir until well mixed, and then brush honey mixture generously on each side of the fillet until fully coated.
4. Arrange the prepared salmon fillets into the fryer's basket, and then fry for 12 minutes until fork-tender, turning halfway.
5. Serve right away.

PESCATARIAN COOKBOOK FOR BEGINNERS

#67 Balsamic Salmon (Instant Pot)

Preparation Time: 5 minutes/Cooking Time: 3 Minutes/Serves: 2 Servings (1 fillet per serving)

Nutrition Per Serving: Carbohydrates: 16.2 grams/Fat: 12.2 grams/Protein: 37.3 grams/Fiber: 0.05 grams/Calories: 325

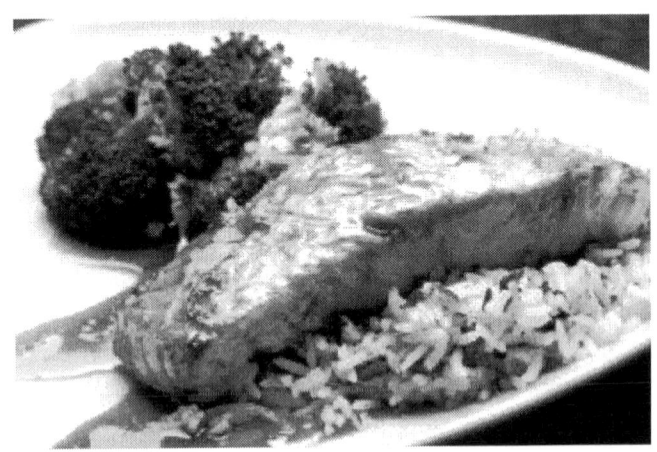

Ingredients

- 2 fillets of salmon, each about 4 to 6 ounces
- 1 tablespoon parsley leaves, chopped
- ½ teaspoon salt
- 2 tablespoons honey
- ½ teaspoon ground black pepper
- 2 tablespoons balsamic vinegar
- 1 cup of water

Directions

1. Get a small bowl, and place honey to it, and then stir in vinegar until combined.
2. Season the salmon fillets with salt and black pepper. Brush the honey-vinegar mixture until thoroughly coated.
3. Switch on the 4-quarts instant pot and pour water into the inner pot. Insert a trivet stand, or a steamer basket, and then arrange prepared salmon fillets on it.
4. Close the cover of the instant pot securely. Press the manual button and select the high-pressure setting. Set the cooking time to 3 minutes, and let it cook. The instant pot will take 5 to 10 minutes to build pressure, and then the cooking timer will start.
5. When the instant pot beeps, quickly release the pressure. Open the lid, and then transfer salmon fillets to a serving dish.
6. Brush the salmon fillets with the remaining honey-vinegar mixture, and then garnish with parsley leaves.

#68 Salmon with Orange Sauce (Instant Pot)

Preparation Time: 20 minutes/Cooking Time: 7 Minutes/Serves: 4 Servings

Nutrition Per Serving: Carbohydrates: 35 grams/Fat: 28 grams/Protein: 51 grams/Fiber: 0.8 grams/Calories: 602

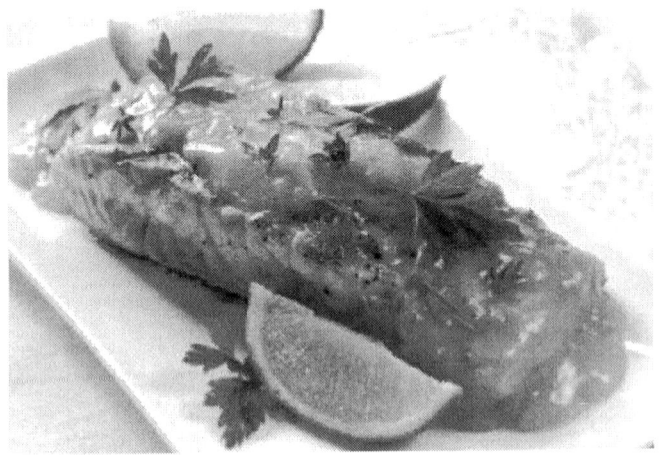

Ingredients

- 1-pound salmon fillets
- 2 cups of water
  For the Sauce:
- 1 teaspoon minced garlic
- 1 teaspoon salt
- 1 teaspoon ground black pepper
- 2 teaspoons grated ginger
- 1 tablespoon soy sauce
- 2 tablespoons orange marmalade

Directions

1. Use a pan that fits in the inner pot of instant pot, or a plastic bag, and then place salmon in it.
2. Place all the ingredients for the sauce in a small bowl and stir until mixed.
3. Pour the sauce over salmon fillets, toss until coated, and then let it marinate for 15 minutes.
4. Then switch on the 4-quarts instant pot and pour water into the inner pot. Insert a trivet stand, or a steamer basket. Place the pan, or plastic bag containing salmon and sauce.
5. Close the cover of the instant pot securely. Press the manual button and select the low-pressure setting. Set the cooking time to 3 minutes, and let it cook. The instant pot will take 5 to 10 minutes to build pressure, and then the cooking timer will start.
6. When the instant pot beeps, release the pressure naturally. Open the lid and then remove the pan from it.
7. Serve immediately.

PESCATARIAN COOKBOOK FOR BEGINNERS

#69 Salmon Salad

Preparation Time: 5 minutes/Cooking Time: 0 Minutes/Serves: 4 Servings (1 salad plate per serving)

Nutrition Per Serving: Carbohydrates: 12 grams/Fat: 16 grams/Protein: 17 grams/Fiber: 0 grams/Calories: 262

Ingredients

- 2 cans of salmon, each about 6 ounces, drained
- 1 medium celery stalk, chopped
- 1 teaspoon dried dill
- 3 tablespoons chopped white onion
- ¼ teaspoon ground black pepper
- 1 tablespoon lemon juice
- 1/3 cup mayonnaise

Directions

1. Place all the ingredients in a medium bowl, and then stir until well combined.
2. Divide the salad in four salad plates or serve the salad in a lettuce wrap.

#70 Caramel Salmon (Instant Pot)

Preparation Time: 5 minutes/Cooking Time: 10 Minutes/Serves: 4 Servings (1 fillet per serving)

Nutrition Per Serving: Carbohydrates: 22 grams/Fat: 30 grams/Protein: 42 grams/Fiber: 1 grams/Calories: 529

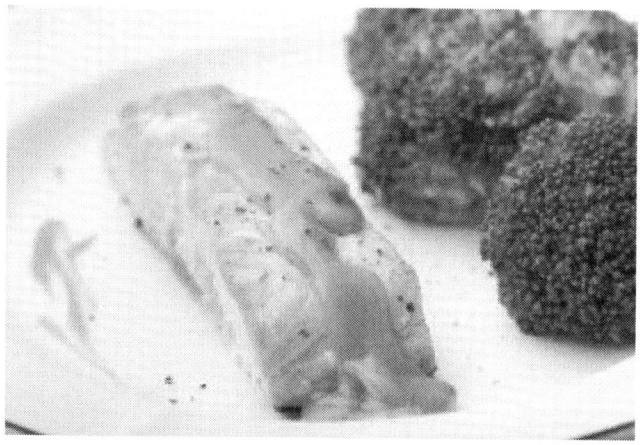

Ingredients

- 4 salmon fillets, skinless, each about 6 to 8 ounces, fresh or thawed if frozen
- 2 scallions, chopped
- ½ teaspoon ground black pepper
- 2 tablespoons cilantro leaves, for garnish
  For the Caramel Sauce:
- 1 tablespoon olive oil
- 1/3 cup brown sugar
- 3 tablespoons fish sauce
- 1 ½ tablespoons soy sauce

- 1 teaspoon grated ginger
- 1 lime, zested
- ½ of a lime. juiced

Directions

1. Place all the ingredients for the sauce, and then stir until well combined.
2. Plug in the 4-quarts instant pot and press the sauté button.
3. Pour the prepared sauce into the inner pot, and bring it up to a simmer, and then press the cancel button.
4. Arrange the salmon fillets in the inner pot (skin-side up). Scoop some sauce over the fillets, and then close the cover securely.
5. Press the manual button and select the low-pressure setting. Set the cooking time to 1 minute, and let it cook. The instant pot will take 5 to 10 minutes to build pressure, and then the cooking timer will start.
6. When the instant pot beeps, let the pressure out naturally for 5 minutes. Then quickly release the pressure and open the lid.
7. Check the fish with a fork if it is tender. Transfer salmon fillets to a serving dish, caramelized side up.
8. Press the sauté button and simmer the sauce for 3 minutes until thickness becomes syrup-like, and then drizzle it over fillets.
9. Garnish the salmon fillets with green onions. Sprinkle with cilantro, and then serve.

Scallops

#71 Scallops with Lemon-Herb Sauce (Air Fryer)

Preparation Time: 10 minutes/Cooking Time: 6 Minutes/Serves: 2 Servings (4 scallops with sauce per serving)

Nutrition Per Serving: Carbohydrates: 5 grams/Fat: 30 grams/Protein: 14 grams/Fiber: 0 grams/Calories: 348

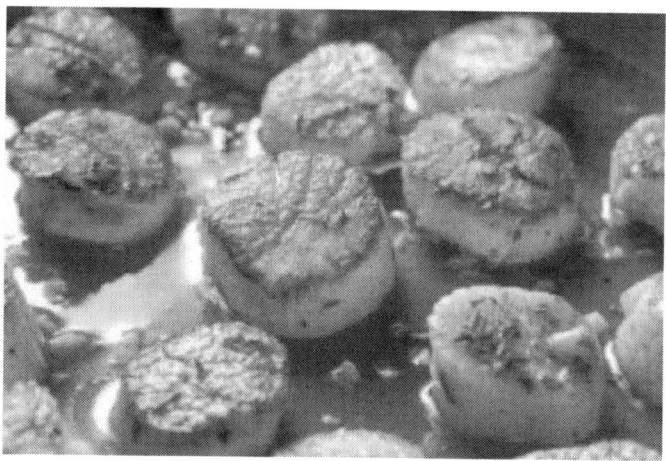

Ingredients

- 8 large sea scallops, each about 1 ounce, fresh
- ½ teaspoon minced garlic
- 2 teaspoons capers, chopped
- ⅛ teaspoon salt
- 2 tablespoons chopped parsley

- ¼ teaspoon ground black pepper
- 1 teaspoon lemon zest
- ¼ cup olive oil
- Non-stick cooking oil spray
- 1 lemon, cut into wedges

Directions

1. Switch on the air fryer and grease the fryer's basket with oil. Insert it into the fryer and close the cover. Select the cooking temperature up to 400 degrees F and preheat.
2. Meanwhile, prepare the scallops. Rinse them well, pat dry, and then season with salt and black pepper.
3. Arrange the seasoned scallops in a single layer and place into the fryer's basket. Spray with oil, and then fry for 6 minutes until done, turning halfway.
4. While scallops' cook, prepare the herb sauce. Place garlic, parsley, lemon zest, capers, and oil in a small bowl. Stir until well combined.
5. When done frying, transfer the scallops in a serving dish. Drizzle with the prepared herb sauce, and then toss until coated.
6. Serve the scallops with lemon wedges.

#72 Teriyaki Scallops (Instant Pot)

Preparation Time: 10 minutes/Cooking Time: 6 Minutes/Serves: 3 Servings (1/3-pound scallops per serving)

Nutrition Per Serving: Carbohydrates: 26 grams/Fat: 6 grams/Protein: 25 grams/Fiber: 0 grams/Calories: 270

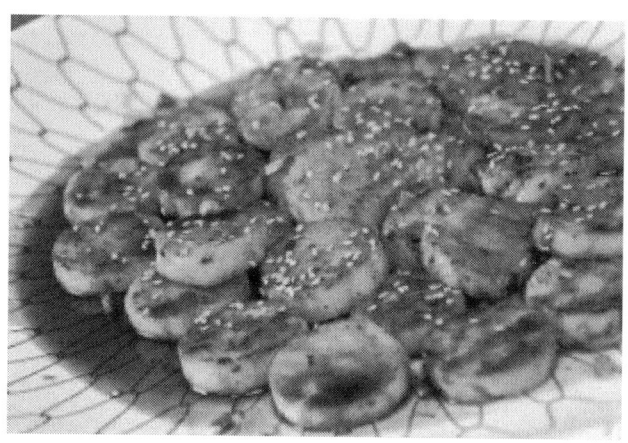

Ingredients

- 1-pound large sea scallops, fresh
- ½ teaspoon garlic powder
- ½ teaspoon of sea salt
- ½ teaspoon ginger powder
- 3 tablespoons maple syrup
- 1 tablespoon olive oil
- ½ cup of soy sauce
- 1 teaspoon sesame seeds

Directions

1. Prepare the sauce. Add garlic powder, salt, ginger powder, maple syrup, and soy sauce in a small bowl and then stir until combined.
2. Switch on the 4-quarts instant pot and press the sauté button. Add oil into the inner pot and preheat.
3. Add scallops, cook for 1 minute per side until golden. Pour the prepared sauce over the scallops and press the cancel button.
4. Close the cover of the instant pot securely. Press the steam button and select the high-pressure setting. Set the cooking time to 2 minutes, and let it cook. The instant pot will take 5 to 10 minutes to build pressure, and then the cooking timer will start.
5. When the instant pot beeps, quickly release the pressure, and open the instant pot carefully. Then transfer the scallops to a dish.
6. Check the sauce and if it is thin and press the sauté button. Cook the sauce for 3 to 4 minutes until it reduced to the desired thickness.
7. Pour the sauce over scallops, garnish with chives and then serve.

NATHALIE SEATON

#73 Scallops with Herb Tomato Sauce (Instant Pot)

Preparation Time: 5 minutes/Cooking Time: 25 Minutes/Serves: 4 Servings

Nutrition Per Serving: Carbohydrates: 25.2 grams/Fat: 8.6 grams/Protein: 37.3 grams/Fiber: 4 grams/Calories: 325

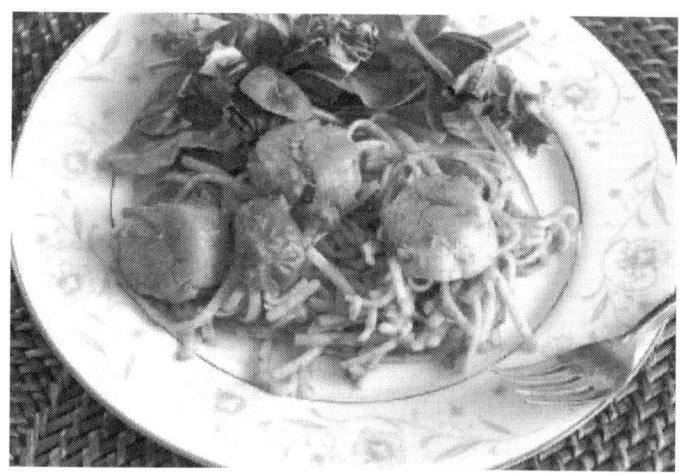

Ingredients

- 1 ½ pound scallops, fresh
- 1 medium red onion, peeled, diced
- 3 ½ cups diced peeled tomatoes
- 1 teaspoon minced garlic
- 1 teaspoon salt
- 1 tablespoon chopped oregano, fresh
- ¼ teaspoon ground black pepper

- 2 tablespoons chopped parsley, fresh
- 6 ounces tomato paste
- 2 tablespoons olive oil
- ¼ cup dry red wine

Directions

1. Switch on the 4-quarts instant pot and press the sauté button. Add oil and then preheat.
2. Add onion and garlic and cook for 4 minutes until onion turns soft. Add tomatoes, salt, black pepper, oregano, and parsley. Pour in tomato paste and wine, and then stir until well mixed.
3. Press the cancel button and close the cover of the instant pot securely. Then press the manual button.
4. Select the high-pressure setting and set the cooking time to 8 minutes. Let it cook. The instant pot will take 5 to 10 minutes to build pressure, and then the cooking timer will start.
5. When the instant pot beeps, quickly release the pressure, and open the instant pot carefully. Stir the mixture, and then taste to adjust seasoning.
6. Press the sauté button, add scallops, and toss until coated in sauce. Cook for 1 minute until sauce begins to simmer.
7. Then press the cancel button and cover the instant pot. Let the scallops stand for 8 minutes until translucent to opaque (Both sides of the scallops should be seared golden-brown).
8. Serve right away, or serve with cooked rice, or spaghetti.

Shrimp

#74 Seafood Gumbo (Instant Pot)

Preparation Time: 5 minutes/Cooking Time: 20 Minutes/Serves: 4 Servings (1 bowl per serving)

Nutrition Per Serving: Carbohydrates: 9 grams/Fat: 12 grams/Protein: 49 grams/Fiber: 2 grams/Calories: 343

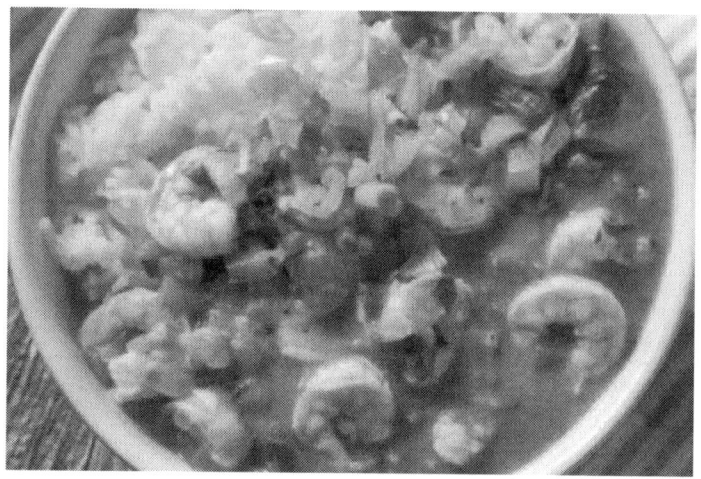

Ingredients

- 12 ounces fillets of catfish
- 1-pound shrimp, peeled, deveined, tail on, fresh or thawed if frozen
- 1 medium yellow onion, peeled, diced
- 14 ounces diced tomatoes

- 1 medium bell pepper, cored, diced
- 2 celery ribs, diced
- 1 teaspoon salt
- 1 bay leaf
- 1 teaspoon ground black pepper
- 2 tablespoons Cajun seasoning
- 2 tablespoons tomato paste
- 2 tablespoons olive oil
- ¾ cup chicken broth

Directions

1. Rinse the fillets, pat dry, and cut them into 2-inch pieces. Season with ½ teaspoon salt, ½ teaspoon black pepper, and 1 tablespoon Cajun seasoning until well coated.
2. Switch on the 4-quarts instant pot, press the sauté button and add oil.
3. Add fish pieces and cook for 2 to 3 minutes per side until golden Then transfer to a plate.
4. Add celery, bell pepper, and onion into the instant pot. Season with remaining Cajun seasoning, and then cook for 2 minutes until fragrant.
5. Press the cancel button and return the cooked fish pieces into the instant pot. Add tomatoes, bay leaf, and tomato paste, and pour in the broth. Stir until combined.
6. Close the cover of the instant pot securely. Press the manual button and select the high-pressure setting. Set the cooking time to 5 minutes, and let it cook. The instant pot will take 5 to 10 minutes

to build pressure, and then the cooking timer will start.
7. When the instant pot beeps, quickly release the pressure, and open the instant pot carefully.
8. Press the sauté button and add shrimps. Stir until well mixed, and then cook for 4 to 5 minutes until shrimps turn opaque.
9. Stir in remaining salt and black pepper and press the cancel button. Scoop gumbo evenly in four bowls.
10. Serve right away or serve with cooked rice.

#75 Shrimp and Grits (Instant Pot)

Preparation Time: 5 minutes/Cooking Time: 30 Minutes/Serves: 4 Servings (1 bowl per serving)

Nutrition Per Serving: Carbohydrates: 22 grams/Fat: 20 grams/Protein: 26 grams/Fiber: 2 grams/Calories: 409

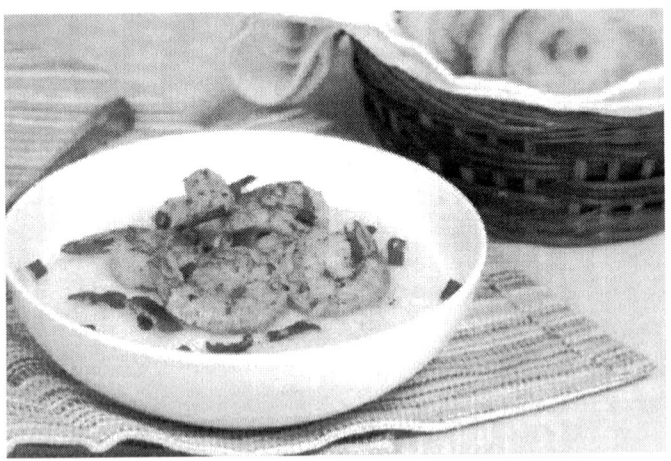

Ingredients

- 1/3 cup grits, old-fashioned
- 4 ounces andouille sausage, diced
- 1-pound shrimp, peeled, deveined, tail on, fresh or thawed if frozen
- 1/3 cup diced onions
- 1 cup diced tomatoes
- 2/3 tablespoon minced garlic
- 1 teaspoon thyme leaves
- 1 tablespoon creole seasoning

- 1 tablespoon butter, unsalted
- 1 tablespoon olive oil
- 2/3 cup chicken stock
- 2/3 cup milk
- ¼ cup heavy cream
- 2/3 cup white wine
- 1 tablespoon fresh parsley leaves, chopped
- ¼ cup sliced green onions

Directions

1. Use a heatproof bowl, add grits, and pour in the chicken stock and milk. Whisk until combined and set aside until.
2. Switch on the 4-quarts instant pot, press the sauté button, and add oil.
3. Add sausage pieces and cook for 5 minutes until the edges turn crisp. Then add onion and cook for 3 minutes until softened.
4. Add garlic and stir until mixed. Cook for 1 minute. Stir to remove brown bits from the bottom of the pot, and then cook for 5 minutes.
5. Add tomatoes and stir in creole seasoning. Press the cancel button, and then insert a trivet stand.
6. Place the grit bowl on the stand, Close the cover of the instant pot securely. Press the manual button and select the high-pressure setting. Set the cooking time to 10 minutes, and let it cook. The instant pot will take 5 to 10 minutes to build pressure, and then the cooking timer will start.

7. When the instant pot beeps, quickly release the pressure, and open the instant pot carefully. Remove the grit bowl.
8. Add butter into the grit mixture, and whisk until combined. Cover the bowl, and let it rest until needed for serving.
9. Press the sauté button, add green onion, parsley and thyme into the instant pot. Stir until mixed and bring the mixture to a boil.
10. Add shrimps, stir well, and cook for 5 minutes until opaque. Stir in cream and press the cancel button.
11. Divide the grit evenly in four bowls, top with shrimp and sauce, and then serve.

#76 Shrimp Tacos (Pan)

Preparation Time: 10 minutes/Cooking Time: 8 Minutes/Serves: 4 Servings (2 tacos per serving)

Nutrition Per Serving: Carbohydrates: 25.7 grams/Fat: 9.7 grams/Protein: 29.6 grams/Fiber: 5.6 grams/Calories: 312

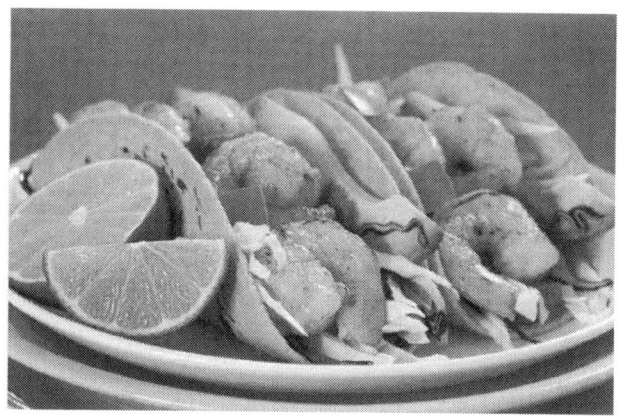

Ingredients

- 1-pound frozen shrimp, peeled, deveined, tail on, thawed
- ½ teaspoon garlic powder
- ½ teaspoon onion powder
- ½ teaspoon red chili powder
- ½ teaspoon smoked paprika
- ½ teaspoon ground cumin
- 1 tablespoon olive oil

- 8 medium tortillas

For the Topping:
- 2 avocados, peeled, pitted, sliced
- 2 medium tomatoes, chopped
- 1 cup shredded cabbage
- 2 limes, cut into wedges

Directions

1. If the shrimps are frozen, rinse them under cool water, then remove their tails. Set aside.
2. Place garlic powder in a small bowl. Add onion powder, red chili powder, paprika, and cumin, and stir until mixed.
3. Place a large skillet pan over medium-high heat, then add oil, and heat until warm.
4. Add prepared shrimps into the pan, and sprinkle with the spice mixture. Toss until well combined, and then cook for 5 to 6 minutes until shrimps turn pink, flipping the shrimps frequently.
5. When done, remove the skillet pan from heat and set it aside.
6. Prepare the toppings, and then evenly divide avocado slices, chopped tomatoes, and shredded cabbage among the tacos.
7. Top the filling evenly with cooked shrimps, and then serve each taco with a lime wedge.

#77 Shrimp Paella (Instant Pot)

Preparation Time: 5 minutes/Cooking Time: 12 Minutes/Serves: 4 Servings

Nutrition Per Serving: Carbohydrates: 39.2 grams/Fat: 9 grams/Protein: 26.8 grams/Fiber: 7 grams/Calories: 315

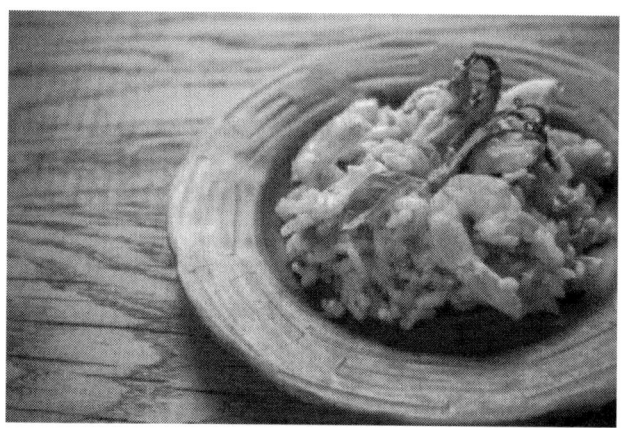

Ingredients

- 1 cup Jasmine rice, rinsed
- 1-pound shrimp, frozen, peeled, deveined, tail on
- 1 red pepper, chopped
- 1 medium white onion, peeled, chopped
- 2 teaspoons minced garlic
- ½ teaspoon salt
- 1 teaspoon paprika
- ¼ teaspoon ground black pepper
- 1 teaspoon turmeric powder

- ¼ teaspoon red pepper flakes
- ½ cup white wine
- 4 tablespoons butter, unsalted
- 1 cup chicken broth
- ¼ cup chopped cilantro

Directions

1. Switch on the 4-quarts instant pot and press the sauté button. Add butter and let it melt.
2. Add onion and cook for 4 minutes until softened. Stir in garlic, and then cook for 1 minute until fragrant.
3. Stir in salt, black pepper, paprika, red pepper flakes, and turmeric. Cook for 1 minute, and then stir in red pepper and rice.
4. Cook for 1 minute. Pour in the chicken broth, and wine. Stir well to remove browned bits from the bottom of the instant pot.
5. Press the cancel button. Top rice with shrimps, and then close the cover of the instant pot securely.
6. Press the manual button and select the high-pressure setting. Set the cooking time to 5 minutes, and let it cook. The instant pot will take 5 to 10 minutes to build pressure. Then, the cooking timer will start.
7. When the instant pot beeps, quickly release the pressure, and open the instant pot carefully. Stir the shrimp paella, and then garnish with cilantro.
8. Serve right away.

#78 Shrimp and Broccoli (Instant Pot)

Preparation Time: 10 minutes/Cooking Time: 10 Minutes/Serves: 4 Servings

Nutrition Per Serving: Carbohydrates: 19 grams/Fat: 5 grams/Protein: 32 grams/Fiber: 5 grams/Calories: 242

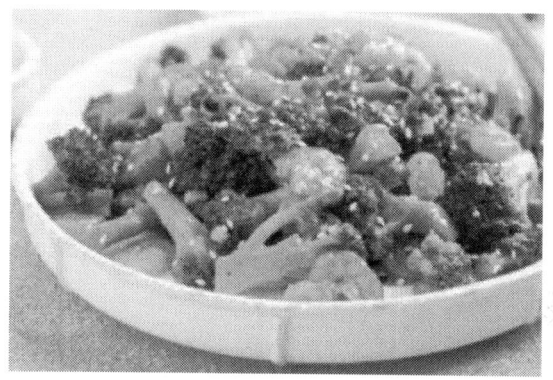

Ingredients

- 16 ounces shrimps, peeled, deveined, tail on, fresh or thawed if frozen
- 28 ounces broccoli, cut into florets
  For the Sauce:
- 2 teaspoons minced garlic
- 2 teaspoons sugar
- 2 tablespoons grated ginger
- 6 tablespoons soy sauce
- 2 teaspoon vinegar
- 4 tablespoons oyster sauce
- 2 teaspoons Sriracha sauce
- 4 teaspoons sesame oil

For the Slurry:
- 3 tablespoons water
- 2 tablespoons corn starch

For the Garnish:
- 2 green onions, sliced
- 2 teaspoons sesame seeds

Directions

1. Place all the ingredients for the sauce in a medium bowl, and then whisk until combined.
2. Switch on the 4-quarts instant pot and pour the sauce into the inner pot. Top with the shrimps.
3. Close the cover of the instant pot securely. Press the manual button and select the high-pressure setting. Set the cooking time to 0 minutes, and let it cook. The instant pot will take 5 to 10 minutes to build pressure, and then the cooking timer will start.
4. When the instant pot beeps, quickly release the pressure release, and open the instant pot carefully
5. Stir together water and cornstarch and add to the shrimps. Press the sauté button and cook for 1 minute until the sauce has thickened to the desired level.
6. Press the cancel button, and top shrimps with broccoli florets. close the cover of the instant pot and let the broccoli steam for 5 minutes until tender crisp.
7. Garnish shrimp, and broccoli with green onion and sesame seeds, and then serve.

#79 Shrimp Fried Rice (Instant Pot)

Preparation Time: 5 minutes/Cooking Time: 18 Minutes/Serves: 4 Servings

Nutrition Per Serving: Carbohydrates: 20.6 grams/Fat: 5.5 grams/Protein: 5.5 grams/Fiber: 0.7 grams/Calories: 175

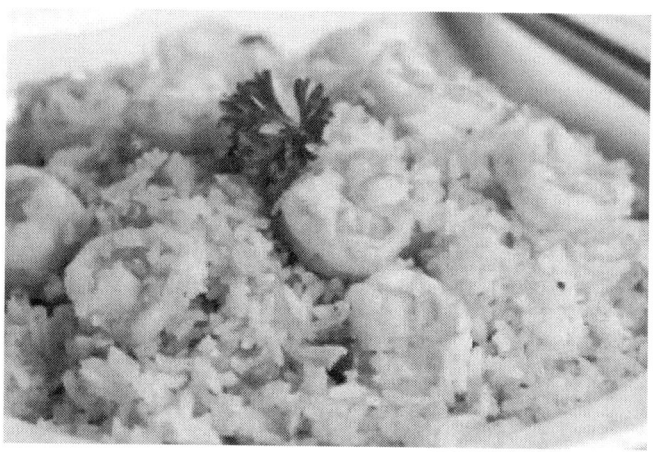

Ingredients

- ½ pound shrimp, peeled, deveined, tail on, fresh or thawed if frozen
- 1 cup long-grain rice, rinsed
- 1 cup frozen peas
- 1 cup chopped white onion
- 1 large carrot, peeled, 1-inch cubed
- 1 ½ teaspoon minced garlic
- ½ teaspoon salt

PESCATARIAN COOKBOOK FOR BEGINNERS

- 3 tablespoons soy sauce
- ¼ teaspoon ground black pepper
- 4 tablespoons olive oil, divided
- ½ teaspoon toasted sesame oil
- 1 cup water
- 2 eggs

Directions

1. Switch on the 4-quarts instant pot and press the sauté button. Add 1 tablespoon of olive oil.
2. Crack eggs into a bowl, and whisk until beaten. Add to the instant pot, and then cook until scrambled to the desired level.
3. Transfer scrambled eggs to a plate. Add peas into the instant pot and cook for 2 to 3 minutes until all the water evaporates.
4. Transfer cooked peas to a plate and add 1 tablespoon oil into the instant pot. Arrange the shrimps in it in a single layer. Cook per side for 1 minute until pink, and three-fourth cooked.
5. Transfer the shrimps to a plate, and then repeat with the remaining shrimps.
6. Add remaining oil, and when hot, add onion and garlic. Cook for 2 minutes until onion begins to soften.
7. Add rice and stir until mixed. Cook for 20 seconds, and then add carrot and shrimps.
8. Pour in water, and season with salt and black pepper. Stir well and press the cancel button. Close the cover securely.

9. Press the manual button and select the high-pressure setting. Set the cooking time to 3 minutes, and let it cook. The instant pot will take 5 to 10 minutes to build pressure, and then the cooking timer will start.
10. When the instant pot beeps, let the shrimps, and rice rest for 10 minutes in warm mode, and then quickly release the pressure.
11. Open the instant pot and add scrambled eggs and peas. Drizzle with sesame oil, and soy sauce. Stir with a large fork.
12. Remove inner pot from the instant pot and place it over a wire rack for 10 minutes, and then serve.

PESCATARIAN COOKBOOK FOR BEGINNERS

#80 Coconut Shrimp (Air Fryer)

Preparation Time: 10 minutes/Cooking Time: 20 Minutes/Serves: 4 Servings

Nutrition Per Serving: Carbohydrates: 23.4 grams/Fat: 9.7 grams/Protein: 12.5 grams/Fiber: 1.3 grams/Calories: 229.8

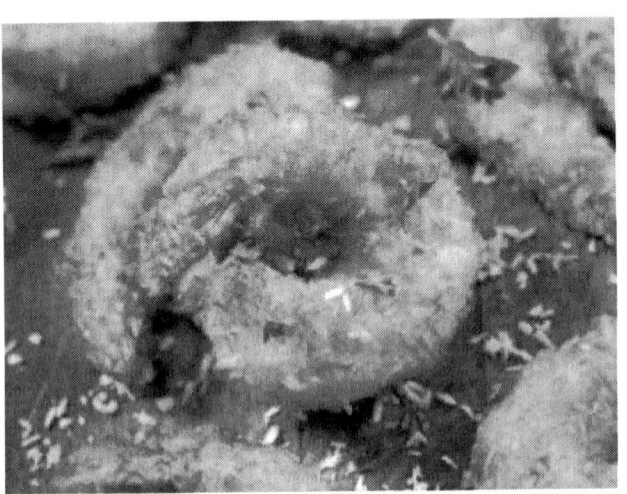

Ingredients

- 1-pound large shrimp, peeled, deveined, tail on, fresh or thawed if frozen
- ½ cup all-purpose flour
- ½ cup shredded coconut, sweetened
- 1 cup panko breadcrumbs
- 1 teaspoon salt
- ½ teaspoon ground black pepper
- 2 eggs, beaten
- Non-stick cooking oil spray

For the Sauce:
- 1 tablespoon Sriracha
- ½ cup mayonnaise
- 1 tablespoon Thai sweet chili sauce

Directions

1. Place flour in a shallow dish. Add salt and black pepper, and then stir until mixed.
2. For another shallow dish, place breadcrumbs, and coconut. Stir until well mixed.
3. Crack eggs in a shallow dish, and then whisk until beaten.
4. Switch on the air fryer and grease its frying basket with oil. Insert it into the fryer and close the cover. Select the cooking temperature up to 400 degrees F and preheat.
5. Meanwhile, work on one shrimp at a time. lightly coat in flour, dip in eggs and then cover in the coconut mixture until well coated.
6. Arrange the prepared shrimps in a single layer in the fryer's basket, and spray with oil. Set the frying time to 10 minutes, and then let it cook until crisp, turning halfway, and spraying with oil.
7. When done, transfer shrimps to a plate, and then repeat with the remaining shrimps.
8. While shrimps cook, prepare the sauce. Place all ingredients in a medium bowl, and then whisk until combined.
9. Serve the shrimps with the sauce.

#81 Parmesan Shrimp (Air Fryer)

Preparation Time: 10 minutes/Cooking Time: 20 Minutes/Serves: 4 Servings

Nutrition Per Serving: Carbohydrates: 12.2 grams/Fat: 16.4 grams/Protein: 27.6 grams/Fiber: 3 grams/Calories: 307.7

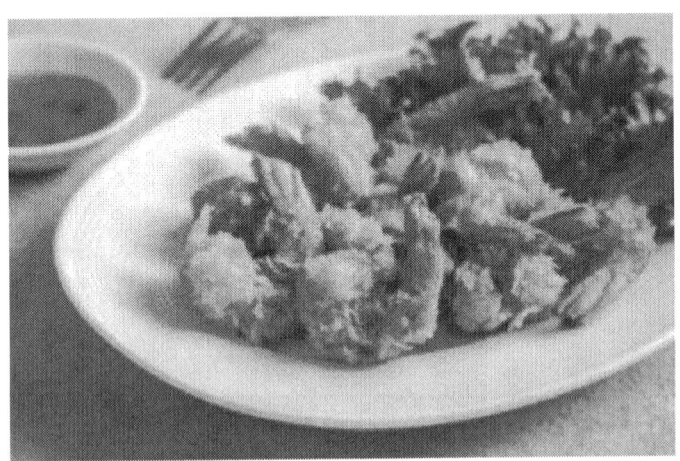

Ingredients

- 2 pounds cooked shrimp, peeled, deveined, tail on
- 1 lemon, juiced
  For the Coating:
- 2 teaspoons minced garlic
- 1 teaspoon onion powder
- 1 teaspoon ground black pepper
- ½ teaspoon chopped oregano
- 1 teaspoon chopped basil

- 2 tablespoons olive oil
- 2/3 cup grated parmesan cheese
- Non-stick cooking oil spray

Directions

1. Switch on the air fryer and grease its frying basket with oil. Insert it into the fryer and close the cover. Select the cooking temperature up to 350 degrees F and preheat.
2. Meanwhile, place all the ingredients in a large bowl for coating, and then stir until mixed.
3. Add shrimps into the bowl and toss until evenly coated.
4. Arrange the prepared shrimps in a single layer in the fryer's basket. Spray with oil and set the frying time to 10 minutes. Let it cook until brown, turning halfway and spraying with oil.
5. When done, transfer shrimps to a plate, and then repeat with the remaining shrimps.
6. Drizzle lemon juice over the shrimps, and then serve.

PESCATARIAN COOKBOOK FOR BEGINNERS

#82 Lemon Pepper Shrimp (Air Fryer)

Preparation Time: 5 minutes/Cooking Time: 16 Minutes/Serves: 2 Servings

Nutrition Per Serving: Carbohydrates: 12.6 grams/Fat: 8.6 grams/Protein: 28.9 grams/Fiber: 5.5 grams/Calories: 215

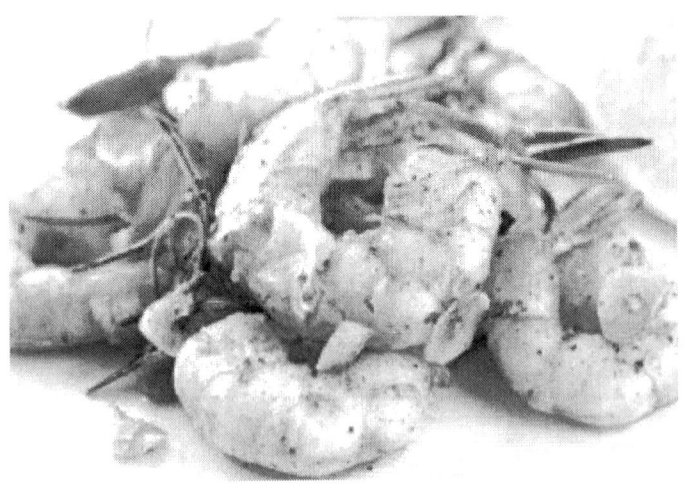

Ingredients

- 12 ounces shrimp, peeled, deveined, tail on
- 1 lemon, juiced
- ¼ teaspoon garlic powder
- 1 teaspoon lemon pepper
- ¼ teaspoon paprika
- 1 tablespoon olive oil
- 1 lemon, sliced
- Non-stick cooking oil spray

Directions

1. Switch on the air fryer and grease its frying basket with oil. Insert it into the fryer and close the cover. Select the cooking temperature up to 400 degrees F and preheat.
2. Meanwhile, add shrimps, drizzle with lemon juice, and oil in a large bowl. Sprinkle with garlic powder, lemon pepper, and paprika, and then toss until coated.
3. Arrange the prepared shrimps in a single layer in the fryer's basket. Set the frying time to 8 minutes. Let it cook until pink, turning halfway, and spraying with oil.
4. When done, transfer shrimps to a plate, and then repeat with the remaining shrimps.
5. Serve shrimps with lemon slices.

PESCATARIAN COOKBOOK FOR BEGINNERS

#83 Salt and Pepper Shrimp (Air Fryer)

Preparation Time: 10 minutes/Cooking Time: 16 Minutes/Serves: 4 Servings

Nutrition Per Serving: Carbohydrates: 9 grams/Fat: 8 grams/Protein: 16 grams/Fiber: 1 grams/Calories: 178

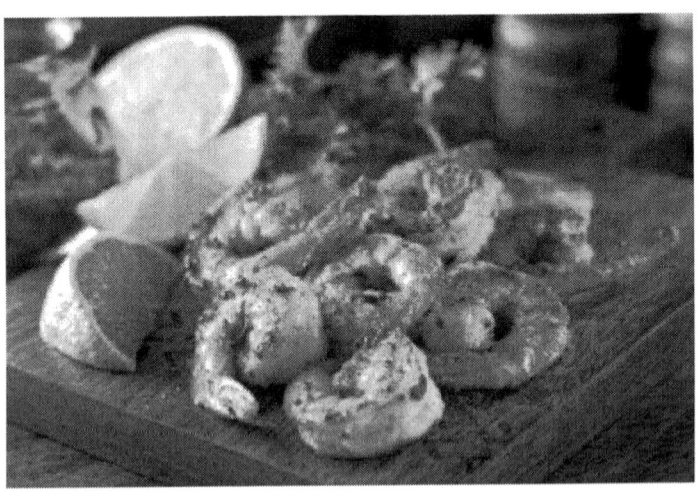

Ingredients

- 1-pound shrimps, peeled, deveined, tail on, fresh or thawed if frozen
- 1 teaspoon salt
- 3 teaspoons ground black pepper
- 1 teaspoon sugar
- 3 tablespoons rice flour
- Non-stick cooking oil spray

Directions

1. Switch on the air fryer and grease its frying basket with oil. Insert it into the fryer and close the cover. Select the cooking temperature up to 400 degrees F and preheat.
2. In a large bowl, add salt, black pepper, sugar, flour, and oil. Whisk until the smooth paste comes together.
3. Add shrimps into the bowl, and then mix until well coated.
4. Arrange the prepared shrimps in a single layer in the fryer's basket. Set the frying time to 8 minutes, and then let it cook until golden, turning halfway, and spraying with oil.
5. When done, transfer shrimps to a plate, and then repeat with the remaining shrimps.
6. Serve shrimps with lemon slices.

PESCATARIAN COOKBOOK FOR BEGINNERS

Squid

#84 Salt and Pepper Squid (Air Fryer)

Preparation Time: 5 minutes/Cooking Time: 24 Minutes/Serves: 4 Servings

Nutrition Per Serving: Carbohydrates: 19 grams/Fat: 11 grams/Protein: 7 grams/Fiber: 2 grams/Calories: 200

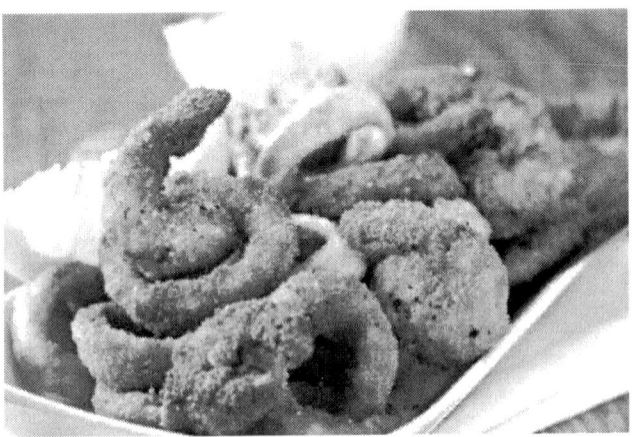

Ingredients

- 1-pound squid, cleaned, cut into rings
- 2 tablespoons salt
- 1 cup all-purpose flour
- 2 tablespoons ground black pepper
- 2 cups panko breadcrumbs
- 1 cup buttermilk
- 1 egg
- Non-stick cooking oil spray

Directions

1. Switch on the air fryer and grease its frying basket with oil. Insert it into the fryer and close the cover. Select the cooking temperature up to 400 degrees F and preheat.
2. Meanwhile, crack the egg in a large bowl, pour in the milk, and whisk until combined.
3. Place the breadcrumbs in a shallow dish. Add flour, salt, and black pepper, and then stir until mixed.
4. Work on one squid at a time. Dip into the buttermilk-egg mixture, and then lightly cover in breadcrumbs until coated.
5. Arrange the prepared squids in a single layer. Place in the fryer's basket and set the frying time to 12 minutes. Let it cook until golden, turning halfway and spraying with oil.
6. When done, transfer squids to a plate, and then repeat with the remaining shrimps.
7. Serve right away.

PESCATARIAN COOKBOOK FOR BEGINNERS

#85 Squid Stew (Instant Pot)

Preparation Time: 5 minutes/Cooking Time: 30 Minutes/Serves: 4 Servings

Nutrition Per Serving: Carbohydrates: 13 grams/Fat: 4 grams/Protein: 27 grams/Fiber: 1 grams/Calories: 218

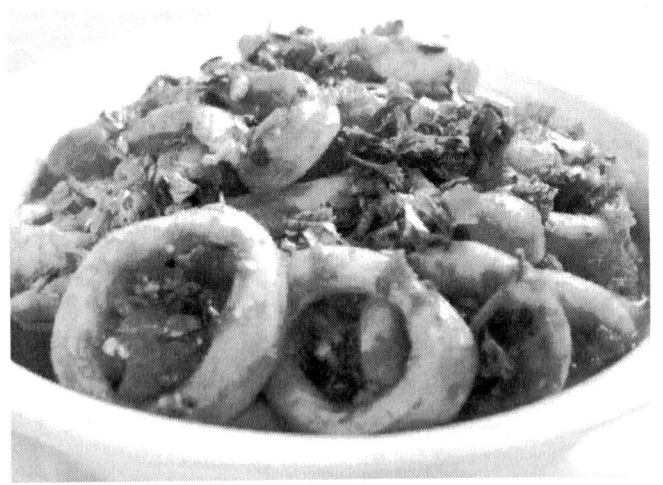

Ingredients

- 1 ½ pound squid, cleaned, cut into rings
- 1 medium onion, peeled, chopped
- 2 cups chopped tomatoes
- 1 ½ teaspoon minced garlic
- ½ teaspoon salt
- ¼ teaspoon ground black pepper
- 1 teaspoon chopped thyme leaves
- 1 tablespoon olive oil
- 2 tablespoons butter

Directions

1. Switch on the 4-quarts instant pot, press the sauté button, and add oil and butter. Heat until butter melts.
2. Add squid rings, cook for 5 minutes until golden brown. Add onion and garlic and continue cooking for 2 minutes.
3. Add remaining ingredients and stir until well mixed. Press the cancel button, and then close the cover of the instant pot securely.
4. Press the manual button and select the high-pressure setting. Set the cooking time to 20 minutes, and let it cook. The instant pot will take 5 to 10 minutes to build pressure, and then the cooking timer will start.
5. When the instant pot beeps, release the pressure naturally and carefully open the instant pot.
6. Press the sauté button and simmer the stew for 3 minutes until slightly thickened. Press the cancel button, and let it rest for 5 minutes.
7. Garnish the stew with parsley, and then serve.

#86 Squid and Chorizo (Instant Pot)

Preparation Time: 5 minutes/Cooking Time: 12 Minutes/Serves: 4 Servings

Nutrition Per Serving: Carbohydrates: 3.1 grams/Fat: 17.2 grams/Protein: 21.2 grams/Fiber: 0.8 grams/Calories: 251

Ingredients

- 1 ½ pounds squid, cleaned, cut into rings
- 2/3 cup diced chorizo
- 2 teaspoons minced garlic
- 1/3 teaspoon salt
- ½ teaspoon lemon zest
- ¼ teaspoon ground black pepper
- ½ cup parsley leaves, chopped
- 2 tablespoons olive oil
- 1 lemon, cut into wedges

Directions

1. Switch on the 4-quarts instant pot, press the sauté button, and add oil.
2. Add chorizo and cook for 5 minutes until chorizo begins to crisp. Transfer to a plate lined with paper towels, set aside.
3. Add garlic and cook for 1 minute until fragrant. Add squid rings, season with salt and black pepper. Press the cancel button, and then close the cover of the instant pot securely.

4. Press the manual button and select the low-pressure setting. Set the cooking time to 1 minute, and let it cook. The instant pot will take 5 to 10 minutes to build pressure, and then the cooking timer will start.
5. When the instant pot beeps, release the pressure naturally, and carefully open the instant pot.
6. Transfer the squid to a serving dish with a slotted spoon and add chorizo and parsley. Toss until mixed, and then sprinkle with lemon zest.
7. Press the sauté button and simmer the cooking sauce for 5 minutes until thickened, and then strain it into a bowl.
8. Serve squids with the sauce.

PESCATARIAN COOKBOOK FOR BEGINNERS

Tilapia

#87 Fish Sticks (Air Fryer)

Preparation Time: 10 minutes/Cooking Time: 20 Minutes/Serves: 4 Servings (4 fish sticks per serving)

Nutrition Per Serving: Carbohydrates: 58 grams/Fat: 7 grams/Protein: 34 grams/Fiber: 5 grams/Calories: 437

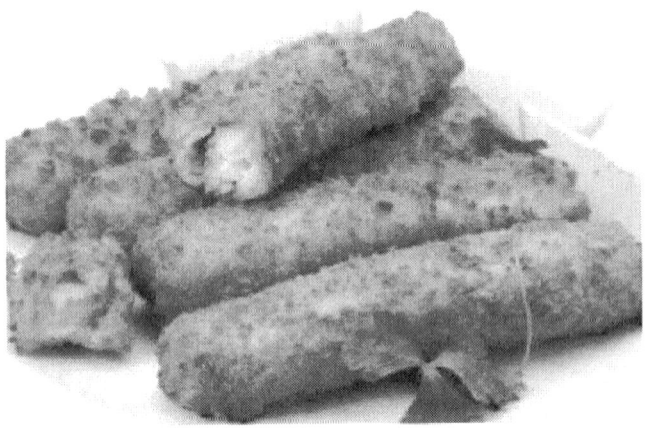

Ingredients

- 4 fillets of tilapia, each about 4 to 6 ounces, skinless, fresh or thawed if frozen
- 1 teaspoon garlic powder
- 1 teaspoon salt
- 1 teaspoon paprika
- ½ teaspoon ground black pepper
- 2 teaspoons old bay seasoning

- ¼ cup whole-wheat flour
- 1 cup panko breadcrumbs
- 1 lemon, juiced
- 2 eggs
- Non-stick cooking oil spray

Directions

1. Cut each fillet into four pieces, about 1-by-2-inches-long, and then pat dry with paper towels.
2. In a shallow dish, place flour, and add salt, black pepper, garlic, and paprika. Stir until mixed.
3. Crack eggs in another shallow dish. Add lemon juice, and then whisk until blended.
4. For the breadcrumbs, use a shallow dish, and then stir in old bay seasoning until combined.
5. Work on one fish piece at a time. lightly coat flour mixture, dip into the egg, and then cover in breadcrumbs mixture until fully coated.
6. Switch on the air fryer and grease its frying basket with oil. Insert it into the fryer and close the cover. Select the cooking temperature up to 400 degrees F and preheat.
7. Arrange the prepared fish sticks in a single layer in the fryer basket, and spray with oil. Set the frying time to 10 minutes, and then let it cook until golden, turning halfway and spraying with oil.
8. When done, transfer fried fish sticks to a plate, and then repeat with the remaining fish sticks.
9. Sprinkle some salt over the fried fish sticks, drizzle with lemon juice, and then serve.

#88 Tilapia with Pineapple Salsa (Instant Pot)

Preparation Time: 10 minutes/Cooking Time: 2 Minutes/Serves: 4 Servings

Nutrition Per Serving: Carbohydrates: 3 grams/Fat: 2 grams/Protein: 23 grams/Fiber: 1 grams/Calories: 124

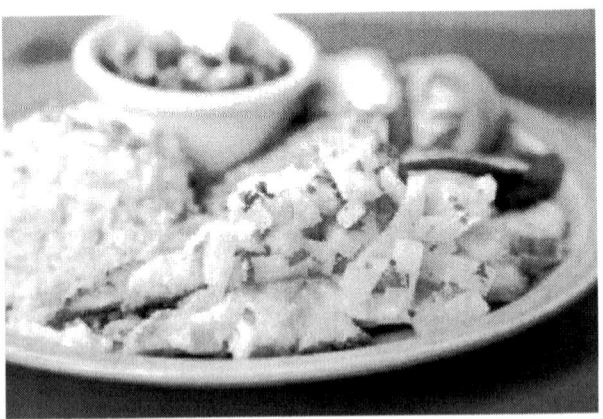

Ingredients

- 1-pound tilapia fillets, skinless, fresh or thawed if frozen
- 1 cup of water
- ¼ teaspoon salt
- 1/8 teaspoon ground black pepper
  For the Pineapple Salsa:
- ¼ cup diced pineapple
- ¼ cup diced tomatoes
- ¼ cup diced bell pepper, mixed colors

- 1 tablespoon chopped red onion
- 1 tablespoon chopped cilantro
- 1/8 teaspoon salt
- 1/8 teaspoon ground black pepper
- 1 tablespoon lime juice

Directions

1. Use a medium bowl to place all the ingredients for the salsa, and then stir until combined.
2. Season the fish with salt and black pepper. Place it in the center of a large piece of foil, and then fold the foil on all sides so that the package resembles a bowl.
3. Top tilapia with salsa, fold the foil over it, and then seal by crimping the edges.
4. Switch on the 4-quarts instant pot. Pour water into the inner pot and insert a trivet stand. Place foil packet on it, and then close the cover securely.
5. Press the manual button and select the high-pressure setting. Set the cooking time to 2 minutes, and let it cook. The instant pot will take 5 to 10 minutes to build pressure, and then the cooking timer will start.
6. When the instant pot beeps, quickly release the pressure, and carefully open the instant pot. Then remove the foil packet from it.
7. Open the foil packet, be careful of the steam. Transfer tilapia, and salsa to a serving dish and then serve.

PESCATARIAN COOKBOOK FOR BEGINNERS

#89 Tomato Basil Tilapia (Instant Pot)

Preparation Time: 10 minutes/Cooking Time: 4 Minutes/Serves: 4 Servings

Nutrition Per Serving: Carbohydrates: 2 grams/Fat: 12 grams/Protein: 20 grams/Fiber: 0.3 grams/Calories: 170

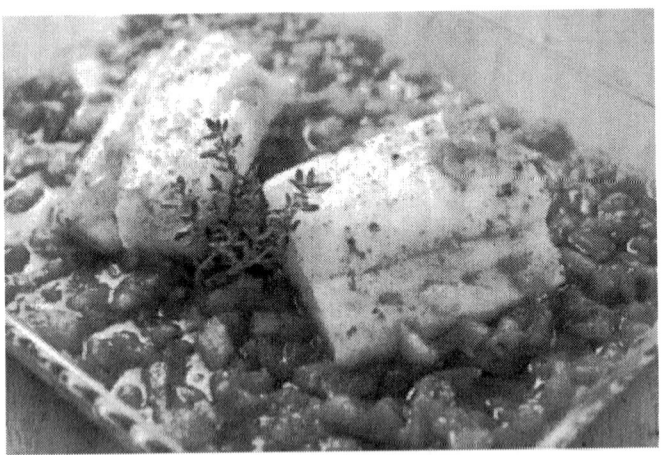

Ingredients

- 4 frozen fillets of tilapia, each about 4 ounces, skinless
- 1 teaspoon minced garlic
- 3 medium tomatoes, diced
- ¼ cup chopped basil
- 1 teaspoon salt
- 1 teaspoon ground black pepper
- 2 tablespoons olive oil
- ½ cup of water

Directions

1. Switch on the 4-quarts instant pot and pour water into the inner pot. Insert a trivet stand, or a steamer rack.
2. Season the fillets with ¾ teaspoon each of salt and black pepper. Arrange them on the trivet stand, and then close the cover securely.
3. Press the manual button and select the high-pressure setting. Set the cooking time to 4 minutes, and let it cook. The instant pot will take 5 to 10 minutes to build pressure, and then the cooking timer will start.
4. Meanwhile, in a medium bowl, place diced tomatoes, add basil, garlic, salt, black pepper, and olive. Stir until mixed, and set aside.
5. When the instant pot beeps, quickly release the pressure, and open the instant pot carefully, and transfer fillets to serving plates.
6. Top the cooked tilapia fillets with tomato mixture, and then serve.

#90 Tilapia Fish Curry (Instant Pot)

Preparation Time: 5 minutes/Cooking Time: 8 Minutes/Serves: 4 Servings

Nutrition Per Serving: Carbohydrates: 6.5 grams/Fat: 8.3 grams/Protein: 22.4 grams/Fiber: 1 grams/Calories: 200.6

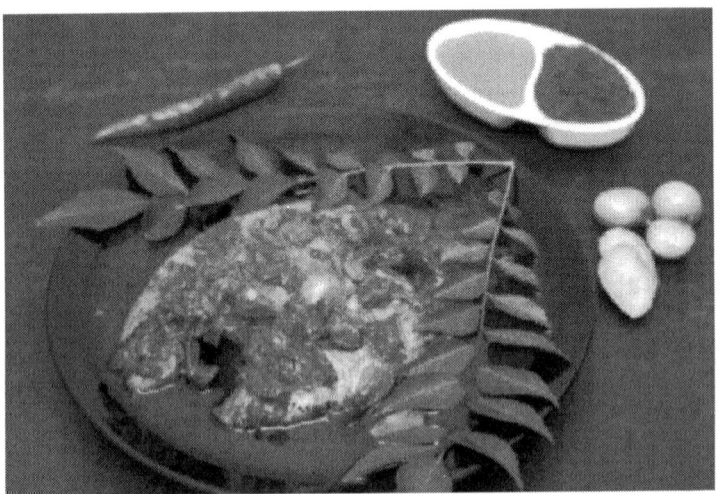

Ingredients

- 1 ½ pound tilapia fillets, skinless, fresh or thawed if frozen
- 2 medium white onions, peeled, chopped
- 1 teaspoon minced garlic
- 1 teaspoon grated ginger
- 1 ½ teaspoon salt
- ¼ teaspoon turmeric powder

- ½ teaspoon cumin powder
- ½ teaspoon paprika powder
- ½ teaspoon coriander powder
- ½ cup tomato puree
- 3 tablespoons coconut oil
- ¾ cup coconut milk, unsweetened
- ½ cup of water
- 2 tablespoons chopped cilantro leaves

Directions

1. Switch on the 4-quarts instant pot, press the sauté button, and add oil.
2. Add onion, cook for 2 minutes, stir in garlic and ginger. Continue cooking for 1 minute until fragrant.
3. Add tomato puree, salt, turmeric powder, cumin, paprika, and coriander powder, stir until mixed, and cook for 1 minute.
4. Pour in the coconut milk and water. Stir until mixed. Press the cancel button, and then close the cover securely.
5. Press the manual button and select the high-pressure setting. Set the cooking time to 2 minutes, and let it cook. The instant pot will take 5 to 10 minutes to build pressure, and then the cooking timer will start.
6. When the instant pot beeps, quickly release the pressure, and open the instant pot carefully. Add fish fillets, stir lightly. Close the cover securely.

7. Press the manual button and select the high-pressure setting. Set the cooking time to 1 minute, and let it cook. The instant pot will take 5 to 10 minutes to build pressure, and then the cooking timer will start.
8. When the instant pot beeps, release the pressure naturally. Carefully open the instant pot and garnish the curry with cilantro leaves.
9. Serve right away or serve the curry with cooked rice.

#91 Lemon Almond Tilapia (Air Fryer)

Preparation Time: 10 minutes/Cooking Time: 10 Minutes/Serves: 2 Servings (1 fillet per serving)

Nutrition Per Serving: Carbohydrates: 14 grams/Fat: 21 grams/Protein: 46 grams/Fiber: 5 grams/Calories: 412

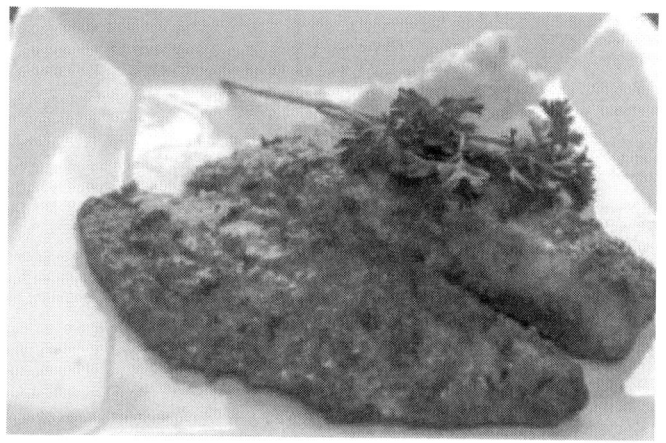

Ingredients

- 2 fillets of tilapia, each about 4 to 6 ounces
- 4 tablespoons all-purpose flour
- ½ cup almonds
- ½ teaspoon salt
- ¼ teaspoon dried thyme
- ¼ teaspoon ground black pepper
- ½ teaspoon lemon zest
- 2 egg whites, beaten
- Non-stick cooking oil spray

Directions

1. Place the flour in a shallow dish, add ½ teaspoon salt and black pepper, and stir until mixed.
2. Place egg whites in another shallow dish, and then whisk until beaten.
3. Place almonds in a food processor, pulse until ground. Tip it into a shallow dish, add ¼ teaspoon salt, thyme, and lemon zest. Stir until mixed.
4. Switch on the air fryer and grease its frying basket with oil. Insert it into the fryer. Close the cover. Select the cooking temperature up to 400 degrees F and preheat.
5. Work on each fillet at a time. Coat lightly in flour mixture, dip into the egg whites and then press the fillets into the almond mixture until fully covered.
6. Then arrange the prepared tilapia fillets in a single layer and place in the fryer's basket. Spray with oil and set the frying time to 10 minutes. Let it cook until golden, turning halfway and spraying with oil.
7. Serve immediately

Trout

#92 Trout with Herb Sauce (Pan)

Preparation Time: 15 minutes/Cooking Time: 12 Minutes/Serves: 4 Servings

Nutrition Per Serving: Carbohydrates: 2 grams/Fat: 24 grams/Protein: 35 grams/Fiber: 0.5 grams/Calories: 380

Ingredients

- 1 ½ pound fillets of trout, skin-on, fresh or thawed if frozen
- 1 teaspoon minced garlic
- ¼ teaspoon salt
- 1 teaspoon dried thyme
- 2 tablespoons olive oil
- 1 teaspoon dried oregano
- 3 tablespoons lemon juice
- 1 teaspoon dried parsley
- 2 tablespoons butter, unsalted, softened
- 2 tablespoons white wine
- 2 tablespoons parsley leaves, chopped

Directions

1. In a small bowl, place salt, thyme, oregano, and parsley. Stir until mixed, and then sprinkle the mixture all over the trout fillets until coated.
2. Place a large skillet pan over medium heat. Add oil, and when hot, place seasoned fillets in it, skin-side-up.
3. Cook the fillet for 5 minutes per side. Remove the pan from heat and cover. Let the fillets sit for 10 minutes until fork-tender.
4. Transfer fillets to a plate. Remove the skin of the fillet. Discard the skin.
5. Return pan over medium-low heat and add garlic. Pour in wine and lemon juice, and then cook for 1 minute until garlic turns soft.
6. Remove pan from heat, add butter and 1 tablespoon parsley. Stir until butter melts and creamy mixture comes together. Scoop the sauce and place over fillets.
7. Sprinkle remaining parsley over the trout fillets, and then serve.

#93 Mediterranean Flavored Trout (Air Fryer)

Preparation Time: 5 minutes/Cooking Time: 20 Minutes/Serves: 4 Servings

Nutrition Per Serving: Carbohydrates: 10.2 grams/Fat: 9.1 grams/Protein: 27 grams/Fiber: 0.7 grams/Calories: 240

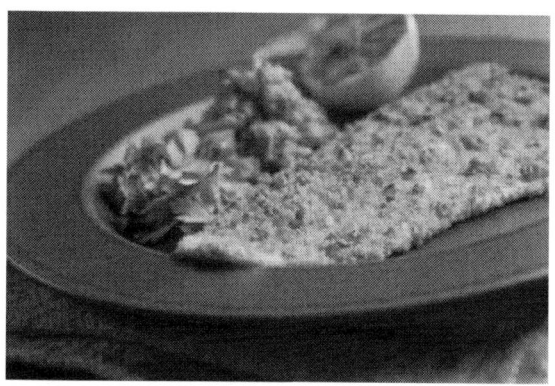

Ingredients

- 1 ½ pound fillets trout, skinless, fresh or thawed if frozen
- 1 teaspoon garlic powder
- ½ cup all-purpose flour
- 1 teaspoon salt
- 1 teaspoon sweet paprika
- ½ teaspoon ground black pepper
- 1 ½ teaspoon ground coriander
- Non-stick cooking oil spray
- 1 lime, cut into wedges

Directions

1. Switch on the air fryer and grease its frying basket with oil. Insert it into the fryer and close the cover. Select the cooking temperature up to 400 degrees F and preheat.
2. Meanwhile, prepare the spice mix. Place garlic powder, paprika and coriander in a small bowl, and then stir until mixed.
3. Season the fillets with salt, and black pepper. Season with the prepared spice mix until coated, and then coat lightly in flour.
4. Then arrange the prepared tilapia fillets in a single layer and place in the fryer's basket. Spray with oil and set the frying time to 10 minutes. Let it cook until golden, turning halfway and spraying with oil.
5. When done, transfer fried tilapia fillets to a plate, and then repeat with the remaining fillets.
6. Serve immediately.

#94 Baked Steelhead Trout Fillet (Oven)

Preparation Time: 5 minutes/Cooking Time: 22 Minutes/Serves: 4 Servings (1 piece per serving)

Nutrition Per Serving: Carbohydrates: 2.1 grams/Fat: 18.6 grams/Protein: 26 grams/Fiber: 0.3 grams/Calories: 280

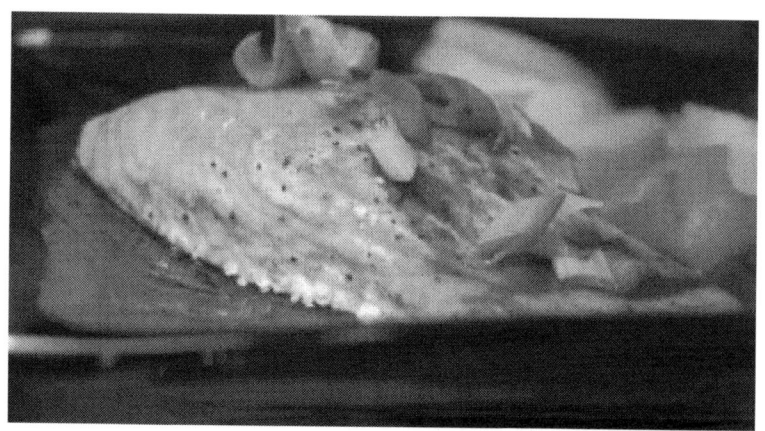

Ingredients

- 1-pound fillet of steelhead trout
- 1 shallot, peeled, minced
- 1 teaspoon minced garlic
- ½ teaspoon salt
- ½ teaspoon ground black pepper
- 1 tablespoon minced parsley
- 1 lemon, juiced, zested
- 4 tablespoons butter, unsalted

Directions

1. Switch on the oven, then set it up to 450 degrees F and preheat.
2. Place a small saucepan over medium heat and add butter. Let it melt.
3. Add shallot, and cook for 3 minutes, or until softened. Stir in lemon zest, and garlic. Cook for 1 minute until fragrant.
4. Remove pan from heat, let the shallot mixture cool for 5 minutes. Stir in half of the lemon juice.
5. Using a rimmed baking sheet, line it with foil, and place fillet on it. Season with salt and black pepper. Scoop the shallot mixture, and then sprinkle with ½ tablespoon of minced parsley.
6. Place the baking sheet into the oven, and then roast the fillet for 12 to 17 minutes until fork tender. Baking time depends on the thickness of the fillet.
7. When done, cut the fillet into four pieces, garnish with remaining parsley, and then serve.

#95 Trout with Chimichurri (Air Fryer)

Preparation Time: 10 minutes/Cooking Time: 20 Minutes/Serves: 4 Servings (1 fillet per serving)

Nutrition Per Serving: Carbohydrates: 2 grams/Fat: 25 grams/Protein: 33 grams/Fiber: 1 grams/Calories: 372

Ingredients

- 4 trout fillets, skin-on, each about 6 ounces
- ¾ teaspoon salt
- ½ teaspoon ground black pepper
- 4 teaspoons olive oil
- Non-stick cooking oil spray
  For the Chimichurri:
- 2 tablespoons chopped white onion
- 1 cup cilantro leaves, fresh
- 1 tablespoon chopped jalapeño
- ½ teaspoon minced garlic
- ½ cup parsley leaves, fresh, chopped
- ¼ teaspoon salt
- 1 tablespoon lemon juice
- ¼ cup olive oil, divided

Directions

1. Switch on the air fryer and grease its frying basket with oil. Insert it into the fryer and close the cover. Select the cooking temperature up to 400 degrees F and preheat.
2. Meanwhile, brush each fillet with oil, and then season with salt, and black pepper until coated.
3. Arrange the prepared fillets in a single layer, and place in the fryer's basket. Spray with oil and set the frying time to 10 minutes. Let it cook, flipping fillets halfway, and spraying with oil.
4. While fillets cooks, prepare the chimichurri by placing all its ingredients in a blender.
5. Pulse until well combined and smooth. Tip the sauce in a bowl and refrigerate until needed.
6. Transfer the fried fillets to a plate and then repeat with the remaining fillets.
7. Serve the trout fillets with chimichurri.

Tuna

#96 Tuna Patties (Air Fryer)

Preparation Time: 10 minutes/Cooking Time: 16 Minutes/Serves: 5 Servings (2 patties per serving)

Nutrition Per Serving: Carbohydrates: 10 grams/Fat: 6 grams/Protein: 26 grams/Fiber: 2 grams/Calories: 202

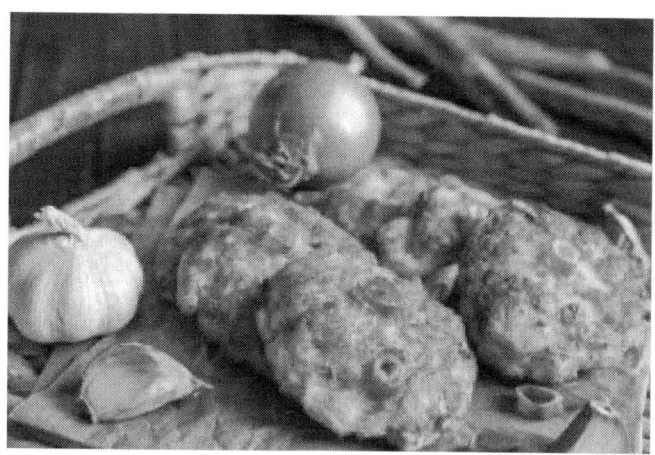

Ingredients

- 15 ounces of canned tuna, drained
- 3 tablespoons minced onion
- 1 stalk of celery, chopped
- ½ teaspoon garlic powder
- ¼ teaspoon salt
- ¼ teaspoon dried oregano

- 1 lemon, zested
- ¼ teaspoon dried basil
- ¼ teaspoon ground black pepper
- ¼ teaspoon dried thyme
- 1 tablespoon lemon juice
- 3 tablespoons grated parmesan cheese
- ½ cup breadcrumbs
- 3 eggs

Directions

1. Crack eggs in a large bowl and add all the ingredients in it except the tuna. Stir until well combined.
2. Fold in tuna and shape the mixture into ten evenly sized patties.
3. Switch on the air fryer and grease its frying basket with oil. Insert it into the fryer and close the cover. Select the cooking temperature up to 400 degrees F and preheat.
4. Then arrange the prepared tuna patties in a single layer and place in the fryer's basket. Spray with oil and set the frying time to 8 minutes. Let it cook until golden, turning halfway, and spraying with oil.
5. When done, transfer fried tuna patties to a plate, and then repeat with the remaining patties.
6. Serve immediately.

#97 Tuna Melt (Air Fryer)

Preparation Time: 10 minutes/Cooking Time: 10 Minutes/Serves: 2 Servings (1 tuna melt per serving)

Nutrition Per Serving: Carbohydrates: 10.1 grams/Fat: 28.4 grams/Protein: 27.1 grams/Fiber: 2.4 grams/Calories: 396

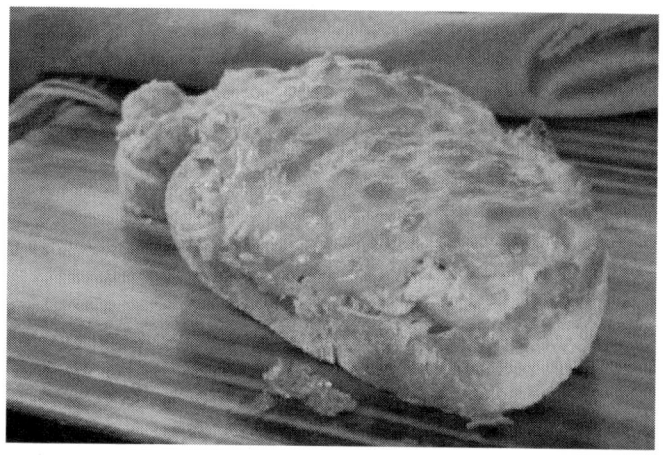

Ingredients

- 5 ounces of canned tuna, drained
- ¼ cup chopped red onion
- 1 dill pickle, chopped
- ¼ teaspoon ground black pepper
- 3 tablespoons mayonnaise
- ½ cup grated mozzarella cheese
- 2 large slices of bread or pita bread

Directions

1. Switch on the air fryer and grease its frying basket with oil. Insert it into the fryer and close the cover. Select the cooking temperature up to 400 degrees F and preheat.
2. Meanwhile, place drained tuna in a medium bowl, add dill, onion, black pepper, and mayonnaise. Stir until combined.
3. Place one piece of bread in the fryer's basket, and then cook for 40 seconds per side until toasted.
4. Then spread half of the prepared tuna mixture on the toasted bread. Sprinkle ¼ cup cheese on top, and fry for 2 to 3 minutes until cheese melts.
5. Carefully transfer tuna melt to a plate, and then repeat with the remaining pita bread, tuna mixture, and cheese.
6. Serve immediately.

#98 Tuna Casserole (Instant Pot)

Preparation Time: 10 minutes/Cooking Time: 1 Minutes/Serves: 4 Servings

Nutrition Per Serving: Carbohydrates: 22 grams/Fat: 8 grams/Protein: 12 grams/Fiber: 3 grams/Calories: 204

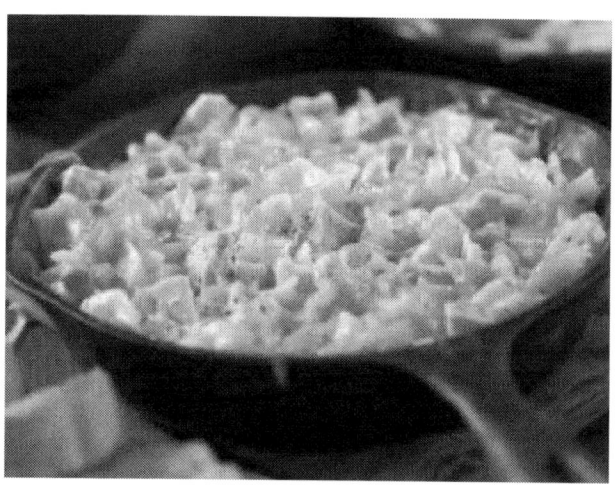

Ingredients

- 2.5 ounces of canned tuna, drained
- ½ cup frozen peas
- 2 whole mushrooms, chopped
- 1 medium carrot, peeled, diced
- 1/8 teaspoon salt
- 1 tablespoon onion powder
- 1/8 teaspoon ground black pepper
- 1 tablespoon milk

- 3 ounces egg noodles
- ½ cup shredded cheddar cheese
- 1 cup chicken broth
- ¼ cup grated parmesan cheese

Directions

1. Switch on the 4-quarts instant pot. Place egg noodles into the inner pot, and then cover with tuna, onion, mushroom, carrot, and peas.
2. Sprinkle salt and black pepper over the vegetables. Pour in the broth and press all the ingredients to submerge them in broth. Close the cover of the instant pot securely.
3. Press the manual button and select the high-pressure setting. Set the cooking time to 1 minute, and let it cook. The instant pot will take 5 to 10 minutes to build pressure, and then the cooking timer will start.
4. When the instant pot beeps, release the pressure naturally, and carefully open the instant pot.
5. Add parmesan and cheddar cheese. Drizzle with milk, and then stir until combined.
6. Serve right away.

#99 Tuna Tacos (Pan)

Preparation Time: 10 minutes/Cooking Time: 3 Minutes /Serves: 4 Servings (1 taco per serving)

Nutrition Per Serving: Carbohydrates: 11.5 grams/Fat: 13.1 grams/Protein: 16.7 grams/Fiber: 1.4 grams/Calories: 233

Ingredients

- 8 ounces of canned tuna, drained
- ¼ cup chopped green onion
- 1 teaspoon lemon juice
- 1 teaspoon olive oil
- ¼ cup mayonnaise
- 4 tortillas

Directions

1. In a small bowl, place green onion, lemon juice, and mayonnaise Stir until well mixed.
2. Place a small skillet pan over medium heat and add oil.
3. Add tuna, and then cook for 3 to 4 minutes until slightly brown. Remove the pan from heat.
4. Switch on the air fryer and grease its frying basket with oil. Insert it into the fryer and close the cover. Select the cooking temperature up to 400 degrees F and preheat.

5. Place one piece of tortilla in the fryer's basket, and then cook it for 20 seconds per side until thoroughly warm.
6. Stuff each tortilla with one-fourth sautéed tuna, top generously with mayonnaise mixture, and then serve.

#100 Tuna Burger (Air Fryer)

Preparation Time: 10 minutes/Cooking Time: 12 Minutes/Serves: 4 Servings (1 burger per serving)

Nutrition Per Serving: Carbohydrates: 35 grams/Fat: 17 grams/Protein: 17 grams/Fiber: 2 grams/Calories: 366

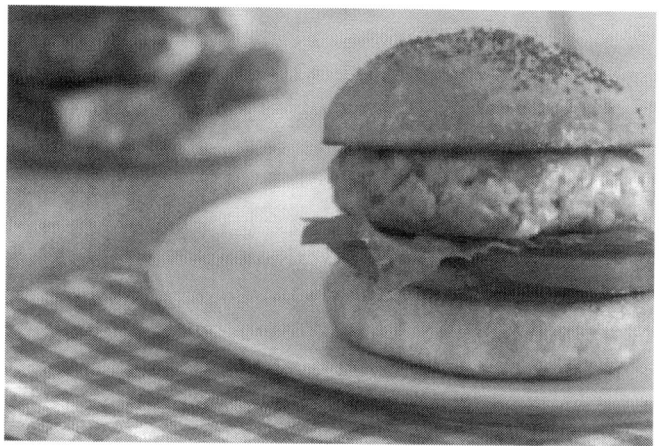

Ingredients

For the Patties:
- 7 ounces of canned tuna, drained
- ¼ cup finely chopped onion
- ½ cup chopped celery
- ½ cup breadcrumbs
- 2 tablespoons red chili sauce
- 1/3 cup mayonnaise
- 1 egg, beaten

For the Burger:
- 4 leaves of lettuce
- 4 slices of tomatoes
- 4 hamburger buns, split

Directions

1. Switch on the air fryer and grease its frying basket with oil. Insert it into the fryer and close the cover. Select the cooking temperature up to 350 degrees F and preheat.
2. Place all the ingredients for the patties in a medium bowl. Stir until well combined, and then shape the mixture into four patties.
3. Arrange tuna patties in the fryer's basket, and spray with oil. Fry for 5 minutes until golden brown, turning halfway and spraying with oil.
4. When done, transfer tuna patties to a plate. Place the bun in the fryer's basket, and then cook for 40 seconds per side until toasted.
5. Assemble the burger. Line the bottom halves of buns with lettuce, and tomato slice, top with a tuna patty, and then cover with the top half of the bun.
6. Serve immediately.

NATHALIE SEATON

Leave a 1-Click Review!

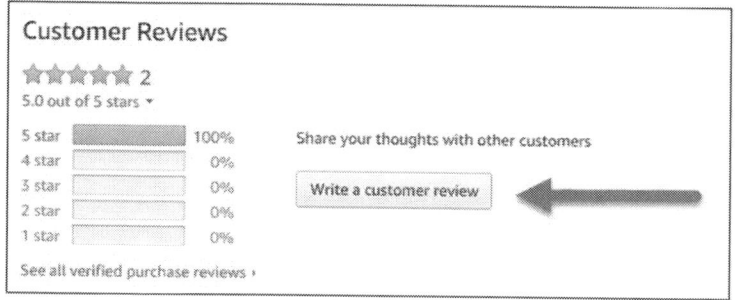

I would be incredibly thankful if you could take just 60 seconds to write a brief review on Amazon, even if it's just a few sentences!

>> Scan with your camera to leave a quick review:

Thank you and I can't wait to see your thoughts.

Conclusion

Cooking can seem like a challenge when you are starting in the kitchen. From picking ingredients in the supermarket to plating the dish in front of your guests, great skill and practice are required. Fishes are no different. Different seafood and fish require different techniques and preparation methods, but if you keep practicing, you will start to commit them to memory. You soon will be able to use them independently without a recipe.

Fish is a great source of nutrition with protein, minerals, and omega-3s. They have noteworthy benefits that are evident in medical tests and have been proven by scientists, comprehensive research, and rigorous trials. Nutritionists and doctors frequently encourage their patients to add fish and seafood to their diets.

Unfortunately, many of us have limited access to good seafood, and when we do, prices are sky-high. It is not your fault that up until now you have not been cooking fish. With this book, you have an array of dishes to choose from that use easy-to-find and inexpensive ingredients. Now, you have no excuses to leave out seafood from your diet. Use the knowledge you have acquired to your maximum benefit.

Once you start making the recipes in this book, you will see visible changes in your health. You will feel more enthusiastic and be less likely to develop life-threatening conditions. There are several meals mentioned in this book, and most are bound to make it on your "favorites" list. Your family and friends will enjoy the diversity at the table as well.

You might think that cooking with seafood will be difficult, so you need to start from the basics to become comfortable. Filleting, deboning, shelling, etc., are not as difficult as some may make them out to be. You just need to keep practicing. There will be some mistakes, but that is normal. It should not discourage you from improving yourself.

So, what are you waiting for? Try one of these amazing recipes today and serve it to your family. Go and add the ingredients to the shopping list if you do not have everything that you need. Begin with something simple and close to your preferences, but try to incorporate other ingredients that you might not use as well. Perhaps, after trying them, you will change your mind.

If you are still sceptical of the advantages of adding seafood to your diet, then try it for yourself and see the results. Do not believe what I say, but instead, give my recipes a test. I guarantee you that they will leave you wanting more. Soon, when deciding what to fix for dinner, the first thing to pop into your head will be seafood.

If you enjoyed reading this cookbook and have gained practical knowledge from it, then leave a positive response on Amazon and recommend it to others. By sharing your experience, you might help others in improving their life.

PESCATARIAN COOKBOOK FOR BEGINNERS

I wish you good luck on your healthy eating journey. I hope that you not only reap all the benefits of eating fish and seafood but that you enjoy preparing them as well.

NATHALIE SEATON

SPECIAL BONUS!

Want These 2 Bonus books for FREE?

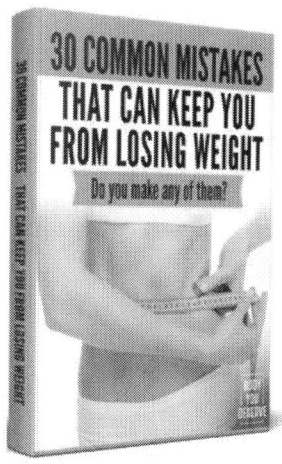
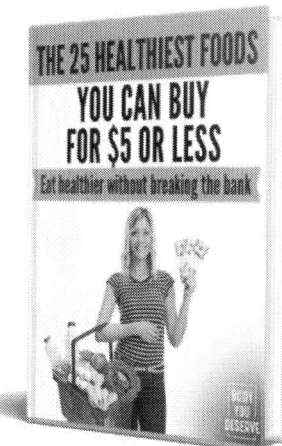

Get **FREE** unlimited access to these and all of our new books by joining our community!

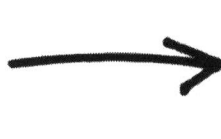

SCAN w/ your camera TO JOIN!

Other Books You'll Love!

Printed in Great Britain
by Amazon